be well assured

be well assured

....

AT THE HEART
of CANCER
THERE IS H.O.P.E.

jen coffel & kim bavilacqua

Published by Advantage, Charleston, South Carolina.
Member of Advantage Media Group.

ADVANTAGE is a registered trademark and the Advantage colophon is a trademark of Advantage Media Group, Inc.

Printed in the United States of America.

ISBN: 978-1-59932-807-2
LCCN: 2016949717

Cover design by George Stevens.

This publication is designed to provide accurate and authoritative information in regard to the subject matter covered. It is sold with the understanding that the publisher is not engaged in rendering legal, accounting, or other professional services. If legal advice or other expert assistance is required, the services of a competent professional person should be sought.

Advantage Media Group is proud to be a part of the Tree Neutral® program. Tree Neutral offsets the number of trees consumed in the production and printing of this book by taking proactive steps such as planting trees in direct proportion to the number of trees used to print books. To learn more about Tree Neutral, please visit **www.treeneutral.com.**

Advantage Media Group is a publisher of business, self-improvement, and professional development books. We help entrepreneurs, business leaders, and professionals share their Stories, Passion, and Knowledge to help others Learn & Grow. Do you have a manuscript or book idea that you would like us to consider for publishing? Please visit **advantagefamily.com** or call **1.866.775.1696.**

I dedicate this book to: God, for instilling an unshakeable desire in me to make an impact on cancer prevention; my husband, Paul, for supporting me in this project and in everything that I do; my four children, Madison, Luke, Lindsey, and Abigail, for inspiring me to learn all that I can to create a healthy home for them. To my dad, Joe Sammon, and my mom, Judy Carney; and my best friend, Jennifer Tessone; I will forever look for ways to honor each of you. —Jen Coffel

With sincere gratitude to: my heavenly Father, for allowing me to live out my purpose and passion; my parents; Penny, Sam, and Dennis for always believing in me and encouraging me to pursue my dreams; and my daughter, Cheyenne. You are my greatest accolade. I love you.
—Kim Bavilacqua

ACKNOWLEDGMENTS

To Jon Evans, the Doer of the Most Important Stuff, who challenged us to write this book. You have been instrumental in helping us create the No Toxin Zone program and our nonprofit, Handing H.O.P.E. You are a gift from God to us, and we are so grateful for all you do.

This book would not have come about without the help of our amazing editor Kristin Hackler. You have an incredible spirit, and we will miss our Tuesdays together.

FOREWORD

"Maybe you should write a book."

Those words were chattering around in my brain after a long prayer session with Jen Coffel and Kim Bavilacqua, so I just blurted them out. This particular prayer session came at the end of what seemed to be a road of tribulation. The three of us had been meeting regularly for over five years to develop an employee wellness program for corporations. At the same time, we were attempting to launch a nonprofit called Handing H.O.P.E., and neither one seemed to be able to pick up any traction. We were stuck, so we turned to our Father in heaven to set us straight.

"Maybe you should write a book." It just kept bouncing around in my head, and as soon as I said it, I could see the look on Jen and Kim's faces. It was that look that mountain climbers get when they reach a false peak and realize that the mountain is way bigger than they had imagined. I felt it too. We had worked so hard for so long, and now this felt like starting over. A book? We have no idea how to write a book. None of us have ever written a book, and we didn't even know anyone who had ever written a book. I left that meeting feeling extremely lost, but by the time we reconvened the following Tuesday, things had changed. We submitted ourselves to God's will and asked Him to guide us and bless the book project. The fact that you are reading this sentence is a testimony to His great power and abilities that go far beyond our own.

I can't imagine a better duo to write a book like this than Jen Coffel and Kim Bavilacqua. They have become like sisters to me, and their godly example of faith in Christ, hope for the future, and love for people battling cancer is extraordinary to witness. Whether you are in the battle of cancer treatments now, a survivor, or simply looking for prevention, this book will inspire, motivate, and move you. The amount of research that these two women have compiled is incredible, and the passion they have to see people make positive changes in their lives is truly inspiring.

It's my prayer that the Lord blesses you with strength and the peace that surpasses all understanding. As you read, I pray that you look for your own personal hope in the stories and testimonies. I would also invite you to do your own research to validate the education, but more importantly, I want to encourage you to make those small changes and take charge of your health. I have seen amazing transformations in relatively short periods of time in my work with a functional medicine practice, and I have witnessed the body's ability to heal if given the right tools. God has a plan and a purpose for your life, and it is all meant for your good. Trust Him.

—Jon Evans, author of *The Doer of the Most Important Stuff: How to Make Better Decisions, Take Action,* and *Get 10 Times the Impact in Less Time*; CEO of Zapaty, a coaching and marketing company; and business director at 3:16 Health Solutions

TABLE OF CONTENTS

INTRODUCTION
BE WELL ASSURED

The cancer crisis is taking a massive toll on our country and across the world. At the time of this printing, cancer is the leading cause of death in twenty-two states, surpassing heart disease.[1]

There is an epidemic of reactionary treatments for diseases in our country. Our current health-care system looks to mitigate the symptoms rather than treat the actual causes. By discovering and treating the source, however, we can not only treat the condition we're suffering from but also proactively prevent so many other potential harms.

This book is written to inspire and educate. We desire to bring hope to those suffering from cancer. For survivors, this book is about staying well by keeping the immune system strong to avoid reoccurrence. It is also for those looking to

---

1 Mike Stobbe, "Cancer Now no. 1 Killer in 22 States, ahead of Heart Disease," Associated Press, January 7, 2016, accessed May 10, 2016, http://bigstory.ap.org/article/4f24b4521c584245b8c7451a503a9ce7/cancer-now-no-1-killer-22-states-ahead-heart-disease.

make simple changes to reduce their risk and enjoy a healthier lifestyle.

In the first part of *Be Well Assured*, we speak to the inspiration that so many cancer survivors have shared with us over the years, either by word or example, as well as our own experiences in overcoming the fear that the word *cancer* can trigger. Most importantly, our hope is that you come away from this book knowing that *there is hope*. Whether it's you or someone close to you who is dealing with this disease, there is strength in knowing that others have traveled this same path and conquered it. In the following pages you'll learn about sources of strength, inspiration, and above all, the value and enduring power of hope.

The second part of this book is dedicated to education, offering the tools and resources you need to implement positive and healthy changes in your own life, regardless of whether you're a cancer survivor or simply looking for ways to proactively prevent so many diseases that are either influenced or caused by the environment we live in.

Cancer has touched our lives in very personal ways. It has led us on a wellness journey, and we have found *hope* there.

Kim's Story

I clearly remember going to the doctor for my follow-up after a biopsy. The fear didn't start as I was sitting with my three-year-old daughter, waiting to be called. It started with the onset of symptoms, the thought of wondering what was wrong. When the results came back, confirming that yes, something looked abnormal and we needed to do more tests, there was fear again as I spent a week waiting for the lab results.

The whole time, I couldn't shake the thought, *Is this it?*

I tried to remain positive, but that nagging fear was never really gone. So I sat in that room, waiting for the doctor. When he did finally call me, he sat down in front of me and said the results were showing that the nodules on my thyroid were cancerous.

I felt as if someone had punched me in the stomach. The air was sucked completely out of the room, and I can't even tell you what he said next. All I could think about was my daughter. As a single mom, I had many thoughts racing through my mind: How was I going to tell my family? Was I going to die? What would happen to me physically? Why was this happening to me?

Somehow, I managed to get my daughter and myself out of the doctor's office and back home, but that terror remained a constant. As the days and weeks went on, there were decisions to be made about treatment options. Then there was the fear of wondering whether those choices were the best ones for my body. Would they work? How would I feel?

That fear was huge, and I know it is for others too. But the good news is that there is hope.

I found my hope in my faith. I prayed, I trusted in God, and I committed to fixing my mind upon living, not dying. On my worst days, when I couldn't get out of bed, God did answer my prayers. He used my illness to reach out to others and share what I have learned on my personal journey, to offer the hope I have found.

There are still days when that fear tries to creep in and say, "Your cancer is going to come back and claim your life." But I immediately recognize that fear is a liar. I continue to trust God for each day that He gives me. I make the best choices I can, based on the knowledge I possess, and I continue to learn more each day on my wellness journey. I am not perfect, but I can do all things through Christ who gives me strength. And I can help others do the same.

Jen's Story

My passion—to bring hope to others—comes from great loss. In January 2013 I lost my dad to lung cancer, and in August 2014 I lost my mom to pancreatic cancer. They were both only sixty-five years old. Then, just a few months later, in October 2014, my best friend, Jennifer, lost her battle with brain cancer at age forty-three. I felt shattered. My grief was almost too much to bear. I needed hope and a reason to go on.

Don't get me wrong. I had many good reasons to live. After six years of infertility, God blessed me with four beautiful children, whom I treasure, and a wonderful, devoted husband of twenty-three years. I also have deep faith, but one of the hardest things about grief is that life does go on. The world doesn't stop. Finding hope in the midst of great grief can be extremely challenging.

My dream is that, out of my loss and all that I have learned, I will be a catalyst for change. I want others to *be well assured* that there are simple steps we can take toward preventing this terrible disease and to know that at the heart of cancer there is indeed hope.

Part I

BE INSPIRED: AT THE HEART OF CANCER, THERE IS H.O.P.E.

"Hope is the only thing stronger than fear."

CHAPTER 1

THE FEAR FACTOR

At the heart of cancer, there is hope, but first, there's always fear. We would be remiss to talk about being diagnosed with cancer and not talk about fear.

Fear begins when the symptoms appear, when you're wondering what's wrong, and the first threads of bright, hot fear begin winding their way to your mind. Then the ultrasound, the biopsy, the nerve-wracking, long wait for results—the whole time you are trying to stay positive, but that nagging feeling keeps entering your mind, and those hot threads of fear are wrapping themselves tighter and tighter.

Then your worst fears are confirmed: cancer. It's as if a prizefighter had appeared out of nowhere and landed a solid uppercut. You can't breathe. Your mind starts swirling with worst-case scenarios, and for some length of time you are unaware of anything but that fact, those words: you have cancer.

That state of shock is different for everyone; how long it lasts and how we handle it are unique to each of us. For many of us, it takes a long time to shake. But when we do, when we start to come to terms with it and realize that we can't live every second in a gripping panic, then we can begin to see it for what it is and realize that we do have options, the first and most important one being that **you do not have to be afraid of cancer.**

If you look at it from a scientific standpoint, not only can you understand it, but you realize that you can do things to proactively overcome it, prevent it, and even eradicate it. That kind of thinking takes away its power. In fact, the nonprofit group The Truth About Cancer created an excellent documentary series on just this subject, which can be viewed at www.TheTruthAboutCancer.com.

The more we are empowered with the truth, the less fear can keep a grip on us. We can annihilate it with knowledge, encouragement, faith, and by taking control of our health by being proactive instead of reactive.

How can we overcome fear?

By knowing that we are stronger than it. Fear is our emotional reaction to danger or the thought of danger. To that effect, some fear is healthy and good. It piques our senses when we are in potentially dangerous situations, such as walking alone at night in an unfamiliar area or when a prowling dog growls at us and bares its teeth. This kind of fear protects us.

It's when we stay trapped in fear, which can create anxiety, that it becomes a self-inflicted poison, crippling us and keeping us from living life.

The Difference between Fear and Anxiety

There is a distinct difference between fear and anxiety, though it may not seem so when you're experiencing either. Both give you that sick, nauseous feeling underscored by low tones of panic. But whereas "fear" is a response to a *known* threat, "anxiety" is a response to an *unknown* or imprecise threat.

Anxiety means you feel uneasy about possibilities. You may have physical reactions such as headaches, chills, or a quickened heart rate, and you may even feel you're losing your mind.

Fear means you have clear knowledge of a definite threat. Your reactions may be the same as they are for anxiety, but you know what you are facing, and from there, you can work out how to face it.

Anxiety eats away at you with every test leading to a diagnosis, and fear sets in when you hear that one word: *cancer*. But in knowing fear, we can choose to acknowledge it and move past it or let it consume our thoughts. The important part is how you choose to cope with it.

There is power in our thoughts. Positive thinking isn't just a mood brightener or a cheesy comeback to someone's negativism: positive thinking has tangible, physical, lasting benefits.

The Power of Thought

In the early 2000s, Dr. Masaru Emoto became known for his famous experiment involving the power of positive thinking and its effect on water crystal structure. Shown as part of the movie *What the Bleep Do We Know!?*, Emoto divided a quantity of water into one hundred petri dishes. Before freezing each one, he would either say something positive to the water or something negative.

The results were breathtaking. The water that received positive words and thought crystalized into remarkable geometric snowflakes, a visual balance of perfection and purity. The negative water, however, either failed to form or turned into awkward, asymmetrical lumps. In some cases, the water even became tainted and sour.

Later, Dr. Emoto tried a similar experiment with cooked rice. He placed the same amount of grain from the same source into three jars, pouring boiling water over each and then sealing them. To the first jar, he would say, "I love you," every day. To the second one he would say, "You're an idiot," and the last one he ignored entirely.

After thirty days, the rice that received endearments had fermented into a lovely, sweet-smelling, early rice wine. The "idiot" jar, on the other hand, had become black and moldy, while the ignored rice was rotting entirely.

It's amazing how much our words matter, not just our words but the intention behind them. Dr. Emoto's experiment demonstrates the visible effects on rice. The rice that heard "I love you" fermented into a beautiful wine. If his words had that effect on rice, what kind of impact could our words with good intent have on people?

As with any study into the power and influence of thought, Dr. Emoto's experiments have received their fair share of criticism, and many people will argue until they are blue in the face that our thoughts have nothing to do with our physical health.

If that's your view, then let us ask you one simple question:

What do you have to lose by choosing to be positive?

Take the story of John Whitley. In 2016, *AARP Bulletin* published an article called "Beating the Odds: Cancer Outliers"[2] that shared some of his incredible story.

At age sixty, John was given less than a year to live. He had been diagnosed with metastasized, stage-four, pancreatic cancer and an inoperable tumor in his liver.

But John didn't let his grim diagnosis take him down. Instead, he signed up for an experimental drug trial in which he was blindly assigned either the drug or a placebo. Along

---

2 JoBeth McDaniel, "Beating the Odds: Cancer Outliers," AARP Bulletin, March 2016, accessed May 10, 2016, http://www.aarp.org/health/conditions-treatments/info-2016/cancer-survivor-prognosis-remission.html.

with traditional chemotherapy, John took his pill every day, and every day he told himself that this pill was the miracle drug that was going to save his life.

Not two months later, a scan of John's liver showed that the inoperable tumor had disappeared, and five years later, John remains cancer free. As for the miracle drug? John had been taking the placebo the whole time.

John's story proves that you have nothing to lose by being positive and everything to gain.

Our friend Jennifer, who was diagnosed with brain cancer and given only six months to live, was a true example of the spirit of positivity.

She could have lost all hope upon hearing her prognosis, disappearing into her fear, but instead, she conquered her fears. Jennifer continued to love people and be an inspiration. She set in her mind that no matter how many days she had left she would be hopeful for healing and live joyfully. Even on her worst days she was thanking others for their help. She made jokes and reassured her friends that she was going to be just fine, and to everyone, including her four children, she was a source of strength.

And guess what? The doctors originally gave Jennifer six months, but she lived three years with stage 4 glioblastoma brain cancer. It was miraculous, and it astounded the doctors. She and many others, including us, attribute it to her positive attitude, to her daily choice to focus on the good, and to express her gratitude for another day. She could have locked herself in her home and been consumed with fear and anxiety, but that wasn't who Jennifer was. She left a lasting impression on many with her courage, hope, and joy. It just goes to show that you lose nothing when you choose to be positive, and at the very least, you gain a positive day.

We all know cancer is life changing. It's inconvenient, uncomfortable, and tests your faith to its core. But if you change your thoughts and focus on the positives, it can have a serious impact on your life and the life of others.

FEAR: Forget everything and run, or face everything and rise.

Surrounded by Survivors

Another way to overcome fear is to surround yourself with those who have already conquered it.

There is strength in knowing that there are other people battling along with you, and there is some camaraderie in going to support groups with others who have cancer, but it's so much more empowering to surround yourself with those who fought the battle and survived. That's where you get your real encouragement.

Survivors are the biggest cheerleaders. They are the ones who say to you, "I know you can do it because I did it. Yes, it was devastating, and yes, it was painful and difficult, and there are days where you just want to give up entirely, but guess what? You can do it if you don't give up!"

But even when you spend every day trying to be positive, and you look on the bright side, there are still days when the battle becomes almost too much to bear and it's hard to find things to be joyful about. On those days, it helps to sit back and take a long, hard look at what you are really afraid of. The reality of fear is this: we are not afraid of heights, but we are afraid of falling. We are not afraid of the dark but rather what's in it.

There will always be days when that fear tries to creep back in, but identifying what we are really afraid of will give us the power to overcome it. In this next chapter, we will share with you some sources of strength we have found that have helped us fight our deepest fears and win.

"You never know how strong you are until being strong is the only choice you have."

CHAPTER 2

SOURCES OF STRENGTH AND STORIES OF HOPE

Any soldier going into battle needs to be strong. It is no different for those in the cancer battle. There are many sources we can draw strength from. Let's start with Hope.

Hope

> *"The human body can live for up to thirty days without food. The human condition can sustain itself for roughly three days without water. But no human alive can live for more than thirty seconds without hope."*

That was the mantra that forty-one-year-old Sean Swarner repeated to himself over and over again after he was diagnosed with terminal cancer at age thirteen and again at age sixteen. Given just two weeks to live, Sean beat the odds and, in doing so, decided that if he could overcome that challenge, he could overcome anything. So with only partial use of his lungs, he decided to become the first cancer survivor to climb Mount Everest.

And he did! Not only did he conquer that peak, but he also conquered the highest peaks on all seven continents, completing what's known as the Seven Summits. He continues to motivate those living with cancer today through his nonprofit, Cancer Climber Association.

Overcoming fear takes incredible strength, and the source of that strength is hope. Strength replaces anxiety—that fear of the unknown—and gives us comfort, which makes a difference not only physically but also emotionally and spiritually. Sean understood the value of hope and embraced it with his whole heart, and we encourage you to do the same.

Care for your mind, body, and spirit by keeping it filled with those things that bring you joy and comfort. It could be as simple as listening to a favorite song that brings you joy or a good book that soothes your spirit. For us, one of our favorite ways to bring peace and comfort to our hearts is with a good, long, honest belly laugh.

Laughter

"Always find a reason to laugh. It may not add years to your life but will surely add life to your years"

It has been said that laughter is medicine for the soul, and we couldn't agree more. Studies have shown that laughter can help reduce blood pressure as well as improve the immune system and increase longevity. If that's the case, then we will live to be two hundred!

What makes you laugh? Think about the last time you laughed until your belly hurt and you cried tears of joy. Maybe it was a funny movie or television show, your favorite comedian, or friends who cracked you up. It felt great, right? You are probably smiling now just recalling it. It's the music of your heart, and every time you let it play, it resounds in every part of you, body and soul. It's a release, and it makes dealing with the hard things just a little less rough. In learning to take life a little less seriously, we learn to see the joy in the simple things every day. For a daily dose of humor about the simple things in life, check out Tim Hawkins on YouTube.

Jen's Story: The Tumble Wig

My mom, Judy, had one of those truly memorable laughs and a beautiful smile.

About three months into her chemotherapy treatments, my mom lost her hair. As you can imagine, hair loss changes your appearance. It kept my mom from wanting to leave the house. She had very limited energy and felt ill often. Easter was approaching, and she wanted to pick out her gifts for the grandkids. To my surprise she put on her new wig, and off we went to Walmart.

When we arrived, I dropped my mom off at the entrance, and as I drove away to park the car, a strong wind whipped through the parking lot and took the wig right off my mom's head, sending it rolling down the asphalt like a silver tumbleweed.

Through my rearview mirror, I watched my mom run after it, weaving her way through the parked cars, but she was unable to grab it, as it was traveling fast! Thankfully, a Good Samaritan caught it and brought it back to her.

I was in shock. I had just seen my mom bald for the first time in my life, and even though the chase only lasted a couple of seconds, I felt overwhelming embarrassment for my mom and began to cry.

When I finally got out of the car and walked into the store, I found my mom sitting on an electric scooter, her wig firmly on her head but very noticeably backward. I didn't know what to do. Should I hurt her pride and tell her I saw what happened in the parking lot and fix her wig? Or should I not say anything and let her ride around the store with haphazard hair?

Fortunately, I didn't have to say a word. When my mom saw me, she started laughing hysterically, telling me all about her hair-raising escapade in the parking lot. She laughed so hard that I couldn't help but join her, and we both just stood there in the store, crying with laughter. When I think about that day, it brings a smile. It is one of my fondest memories.

When confronted with the choice of whether to laugh or cry, choosing to laugh can be powerful. By opening up and embracing the joy of a moment, you are giving yourself a solid dose of the best mental and physical medicine there is: laughter.

Change of Scenery

"Sometimes, you just need a break. In a beautiful place. Alone. To figure everything out."

When the pressure starts to build, we like to head to the beach. It's so peaceful to sit on the shore, listen to the slow hush and roll of the waves, soak in the sunlight, and let any cares and worries melt away. For others, the place of peace may be in the mountains, traveling to distant lands, or just stretching out in a lawn chair by a lake or in the backyard.

Changes of scenery give us a break from reality, even if only for a moment. These small breaks help us reenergize and get a fresh perspective on the world. In a way, it's kind of like a grown-up time-out that we can look forward to!

And a time-out was exactly what Julie needed.

After going through a bilateral mastectomy and twelve weeks of chemotherapy, Julie needed a change of scenery. She sought solace at a friend's lakeside cabin and would spend hours simply staring across the lake, soaking in the peace and beauty of nature.

It was during that time of quiet restoration that she began thinking of ways she could give back to her community and support other survivors. She wanted to spread the message of courage, strength, and hope that had supported her through those long months of treatment and recovery and found that she could do that through her art.

As her physical strength grew, so did her spiritual strength as she began expressing herself through art, and soon she was encouraging others to do the same, helping them create the scenery that most empowered them through the art medium of their choice as they bravely walked the road to recovery.

Where do you like to go for a change of scenery when you need to gain a fresh perspective?

Music

"Music washes away from the soul the dust of everyday life."

Music can be a huge source of comfort. Just as music soothes the savage beast, it also soothes the savage soul. When you are overwrought with anxiety, sometimes the best thing you can do for yourself is sit down, take a deep breath, and turn on some music that brings you peace and comfort. It could be a calming instrumental piece or lyrics that speak of strength, peace, and joy. The best inspirational music is both heard and felt, sometimes bringing us to healthy tears as we release our pent-up emotions and other times inspiring us to leap out of our seats and sing at the top of our lungs as though no one is listening or dance as if no one is watching. Just letting yourself be in the moment and be swept away by song can be an incredible and invigorating experience!

The *Comfort CD* by Kathy Troccoli is a great source of inspiration for those battling cancer and their families. Kathy Troccoli was fifteen when she lost her father to colon cancer and thirty-three when she lost her mother to breast cancer. In an interview with Christian Broadcasting Network shortly after her album came out in 2005,[3] Kathy said, "What I have found is [that] a four-minute song can do more than any book or sermon. It's just powerful." She added, "I've gone through my own sorrows in life—music has been able to penetrate the darkness . . . I wanted to do a record that you could play all the way through and have it be like a healing balm for your soul."

Her music has been a great source of comfort, and it has truly served as a soothing balm for many people in dark and difficult times.

Literature

> *"The reading of all good books is like a conversation with the finest minds of past centuries." -Rene Descartes*

A good book is a great escape. Whether you go for an e-book, an audiobook, or a good old-fashioned paperback, there is

---

3 "You've Got a Friend in Kathy Troccoli," Christian Broadcast Network, accessed May 10, 2016, http://www1.cbn.com/music/you%26rsquo%3Bve-got-a-friend-in-kathy-troccoli.

plenty of wonderful literature to choose from that can offer strength and encouragement and a much-needed romp through the imagination.

One of our favorite stories of hope and inspiration comes from the book *Open Your Eyes* by Jake Olson and McKay Christiansen.

JAKE OLSON'S STORY

At only a few months old, Jake Olson was diagnosed with a very rare childhood cancer, retinal blastoma, which affects the inner lining of the eye. Because of this, his left eye had to be removed when he was ten months old and, due to the extreme nature of the cancer, his right eye also needed to be removed when he was twelve.

The night before his second surgery, Jake got to enjoy one of his favorite activities: football. His parents took him to a University of Southern California (USC) football practice, and for a while, Jake put aside thoughts of the surgery he would have to undergo the next day. But on the way home, Jake suddenly realized that this would be the last time he would see the outside world. He desperately pressed his nose to the window, taking in everything he could as tears streamed down his face. It broke his parents' hearts to watch him.

Jake came out of his surgery the next day with an amazingly bright attitude. He wasn't sad, only relieved that the surgery was finally over and he could get on with life.

It was incredible for his family and friends to see such a strong, positive attitude in one so young, and that strength of character has carried Jake to some amazing places.

Not five days after his surgery, Jake was playing football, drawing from his memories of watching the game being played and relying on his quickly sharpening sense of hearing. In fact, this talent led the USC football team to bring him on as a long snapper once he graduated high school.

And he's not limiting himself to just one sport. Jake also hopes to one day be the first blind person to play in the Professional Golfers Association (PGA). He also enjoys skiing and surfing.

Today Jake has developed many talents, and he tours as a motivational speaker, speaking at schools and local events as well as making national broadcasts for media such as ESPN and *Katie*. His foundation, Out of Sight Faith, continues to grow as it provides blind children with much-needed support and resources.

In his book *Open Your Eyes*, which he coauthored at age sixteen with Dr. McKay Christensen, Jake states:

> My courage, my strength and my perseverance all start with my faith . . . [God] is the reason I wake up every day with hope and confidence for what that day will bring . . . Knowing God is in control and that He loves me give me great peace. Psalm 29:11 states, "The Lord gives strength to his people; the Lord blesses His people with peace"

I [also] put complete trust in Jeremiah 29:11: "'For I know the plans I have for you,' declares the Lord, 'plans to prosper you and not to harm you, plans to give you a hope and a future.'" It gives me encouragement and hope, and it has helped me get though some of the most difficult times and challenges.

Hope is my foundation, and it helped me get through a lot of dark days.

It's so inspiring to us how Jake has dealt with the loss of his sight. Despite being unable to see, he still has amazing vision: vision of strength and hope and of living life to its fullest, accepting and conquering the challenges he faces along the way.

When we think about Jake, overcomer is what comes to mind. He truly inspires us and is a great example that anything is possible.

Here are some other inspirational readings we recommend:

- *Jesus Calling* by Sarah Young
- *Imagine Heaven* by John Burke
- *The Survivors Club* by Ben Sherwood
- *Messages of Hope* by Duane Zavaya
- *Dying to Be Me* by Anita Moorjani

Physical Touch

"Touch comes before sight, before speech. It is the first language, and the last, and it always tells the truth" - Margaret Atwood

So many of us are comforted by physical touch. When a baby cries, our first reaction is to pick it up and rock it until it calms down and is comforted. The same is true of adults. Hugs, handholding, and even a gentle hand placed on a shoulder can bring an incredible amount of comfort to someone in need of that all-too-important human connection.

Massage is a great example of this. Many people, including cancer survivors, have shared with us how extremely therapeutic massage can be. It can release toxins, promote total relaxation, and relieve pain associated with symptoms. It can break up scar tissue and help with postsurgical swelling. In fact, a study published in 2013 in *Applied Nursing Research* compared twenty patients who received back massages during chemotherapy to twenty who did not. The researchers found that massage helped reduce anxiety and fatigue during and after chemotherapy—even the mind benefits from it. Massage relaxes and helps all that stress fade away.[4] Many would agree massage is a necessity disguised as a luxury.

---

4 Serife Karagozoglu et al., "Effects of Back Massage on Chemotherapy-Related Fatigue and Anxiety: Supportive Care and Therapeutic Touch in Cancer Nursing," *Applied Nursing Research* 26, no. 4: 210–217.

Gratitude

"Gratitude turns what we have into enough, and more. It turns denial into acceptance, chaos into order, confusion into clarity...it makes sense of our past, brings peace for today, and creates a vision for tomorrow." - Melody Beattie

Gratitude is one of those rare things that you get more of by giving away.

Naming the things we are grateful for puts our focus on the positives we have in life and takes it off of the negatives. Some of us journal or keep sticky notes around mirrors or come up with any number of creative little ways to remember what we are grateful for. Gratitude journals are helpful for those of us who find strength in writing down what we are grateful for every day. It teaches us thankfulness and keeps our thoughts in a positive place.

Gratitude stifles the dark voice of illness that whispers to us, insisting that all we have become is our disease.

A WORD FROM JEN

My best friend, Jennifer, was a great example of living with gratitude. She left a legacy of gratitude that has forever left an imprint on my heart. She was a huge inspiration and source of strength as I struggled with the loss of my mom and dad to cancer. As her power of medical attorney, I attended almost every single doctor appointment with her for three years. During that time, she ended up having three craniotomies.

The first one was the scariest. The brain tumor was so large that she was having difficulty speaking, and her memory loss was quickly worsening. Due to the severity and size of the tumor, the surgeons were unable to do brain mapping to locate the speech and memory centers of her brain tissue prior to surgery. They were very concerned that she would lose her memory and her ability to speak after surgery, which deeply concerned me. *Even if my friend survives this surgery,* I thought, *would she still be the same Jennifer?*

I was the first to see her in recovery, and I had no idea what to expect. From the hallway, I could hear her getting sick from the anesthesia, and when I walked into the room, I found her hanging over the hospital rail in tremendous pain.

But when she saw me standing by her bedside, she smiled and said, "Thank you, Jen," as clearly as could be.

I began laughing and crying at the same time and realized that my prayers had been answered, and my best friend not only remembered me but could also speak.

That day, Jennifer taught me a life lesson that I will never forget about thankfulness: even in the midst of great pain and suffering, she could smile and express gratitude.

Meditation and Prayer

"Lord, help me trust you and your perfect plan. Quiet the fears in my spirit. I surrender my life to you now, in Jesus's name."

Jen's dad, Joe, wrote this prayer before he passed away. For Jen, it was a simple yet powerful prayer that gave her complete peace and reassured her that she would see him again in heaven.

Prayer and/or meditation are incredibly valuable for lots of people, including us. Daily meditation on God's word and conversations with God can bring clarity, comfort, and peace. Being able to express ourselves in these private, focused moments helps to fill our hope tanks. Whether it's an affirmation that brings us that particular peace or a Bible verse that encourages us in times of distress, prayer can bring healing and hope for the future.

For those who look to God, faith becomes a phenom-enal source of strength. Faith allows us to trust in things we cannot see. It lets us know that we aren't alone on life's journey, that someone greater than us can sustain us if we put our trust and hope in Him. This faith is what brings us the ultimate sense of peace.

Rebecca's incredible story is about the power of prayer for healing. At age sixty, Rebecca was diagnosed with thyroid cancer. One week before her scheduled surgery, Rebecca and her husband went to the elders of their church and prayed together. Miraculously, after her surgery, Rebecca's biopsy showed that her thyroid was completely cancer free! Rebecca had the courage and audacious faith to ask and trust God for healing. She received that miracle through the power of prayer.

Sometimes we do not know how or what to pray for a loved one. This is how we pray for a friend or family member who is ill:

Lord, your word speaks promises of healing and restoration. I thank you for the miracles you still perform today. Today I claim those promises over [my friend's name]. I believe in your healing power. I ask you to begin your mighty work in the life of [my friend's name]. Please surround [my friend's name] with supernatural peace and strength and give [my friend's name] the faith to believe that all things are possible through you. Protect [my friend's name] from discouragement, and let miraculous healing begin. Amen.

When we are overwhelmed or afraid, we don't always know how to pray for our own healing. If you are battling cancer, here is a prayer of healing:

God, you know me so well. You created me. You know the number of hairs on my head, and you even know the thoughts conceived in my heart before I ever vocalize them. You've told us to come to you and ask for every need of life. I'm coming to you today and asking for your divine healing. There's so much I don't understand about life. But I do know that with one touch, one word, you can make me whole. Please forgive me of my sins and begin your healing from the inside out. I don't always know what your will is, Lord, especially in times like now. I simply bow my heart before you to tell you if you choose to use doctors to provide healing, give them wisdom to know what to do. Regardless of how you accomplish it, the healing you give is always miraculous. And you deserve all the praise. Ultimately, I want your will to be my will. Use this trial to strengthen me from a what-if faith to a no-matter-what faith. And no matter what, I choose to know your grace is sufficient and your plan is perfect. In Jesus's name, amen.

There is power in prayer, in being able to take that great burden of worry and pain and place it in His hands. And in His peace, we find our own. Being in that place of peace is where we surrender our fear and also visualize our healing.

Visualization

"Visualization is daydreaming with a purpose."

The practice of visualization can be powerful. On its own, visualization provides the comfort of picturing yourself where you want to be, feeling the way you want to feel, and living the way you want to live. Visualize yourself healthy, strong, and joyful, and you take the power away from feelings of sadness and defeat. If you refuse to see yourself as sick, as a victim, then you're giving yourself the power to not only believe you are stronger but also to *be* stronger.

In the morning, before your feet hit the ground, visualize your ideal day. Then at night, before you go to bed, do the same for the next day. What does it look and feel like? Really spend time formulating your thoughts. It may seem awkward at first, but these brief moments of focus at the edges of the day draw the subconscious mind into the forefront and allow you to begin moving toward those things naturally.

At the same time, your physical living space should also reflect feelings of peace and happiness. A dark, cluttered, dirty room will only lead to similar thoughts. But a clean room filled with light and pictures of loved ones and/or places that have brought you peace and happiness will help you feel the same.

CREATE A VISION BOARD

Vision boards are an easy, beautiful way to keep all the things that mean the most to you front and center in your thoughts. They can be made from anything—from poster board to corkboard to old picture frames—and should include all the things that bring joy to your life, from family photos to magazine clippings of faraway places. The purpose is for those pictures and words to bring life to what you desire today and in the future. The board is a snapshot of your perceived future and your desires.

Be Purposeful

"Your life won't ever be perfect, but it can be purposeful. Live for something bigger than yourself and leave a mark on the world."

Regardless of what it is you do to bring strength, hope and peace to your life, the important thing is to do it with purpose. Everyone is different, but whether you believe that laughing, listening to music, praying, reading, or traveling is what will bring you strength, then you should take action on it. Choose to be strong and do it with purpose!

Wanda Draus's story is a great example of being purposeful. Out of her own cancer battle came her nonprofit Basket of Courage. This is her story.

WANDA'S STORY

It was a chilly morning as Wanda waited for her teapot to whistle, the day as overcast as her soul felt. It had been two long days since her biopsy, and she was still waiting for an answer.

Truly, with something this important, they would call me right away, she thought, reminding herself that no news was good news.

But on the third day, after leaving an inquiring message with her doctor's answering service, Wanda got the call. At first she was relieved to hear her doctor's voice, but nothing prepared her for what she said.

"You have breast cancer, invasive ductal carcinoma," she told Wanda.

Wanda didn't really hear the doctor's next words. As her doctor began to talk about next steps, scheduling tests and choosing a team, Wanda kept hearing, "You have breast cancer." It was with a shaky hand that she began taking notes, the doctor rattling off something about limited treatment, aggressive, triple negative—but it was all difficult to comprehend.

"I don't remember hanging up the phone. I just remember being alone, and I couldn't stop my body from shaking," Wanda said. "I made my way to the bedroom, lay across the bed, and for the first time, felt tremendous fear. Even through the difficult times in my life—divorce, financial struggle, being a single mom to teenage boys—nothing gripped me like this. I always knew God was there through every trial, through every blessing, but what happened here? Why was I filled with such fear?"

Tears ran down Wanda's face as questions whirled through her mind. How was she going to tell her family, her husband? What had she done or not done to deserve this?

Despite her fear, Wanda still felt God's peace and reached out to him in prayer.

"I asked God if this was a trial for someone else to know Him, and if so, couldn't there have been another way?" Wanda said.

As those thoughts swept over her, Wanda felt a stillness in the room, and it was suddenly as if Christ were sitting at the end of her bed and reminding her, "I had to die on a cross for you to know me because there was no other way."

Wanda had to endure months of surgeries, setbacks, chemotherapy, and radiation, but the love and support from her friends, family, and even strangers inspired her to keep fighting, and God's word kept her strong.

"The fear that was trying to paralyze me and take away my joy was replaced with a deeper and stronger faith that I'm in God's hands no matter the outcome," Wanda said.

On her last day of treatment, she took all of the beautiful cards that people had sent to her over the months, tied a pink ribbon around them, and packed them away. That day, she said to herself she was done with tests, done with hospitals, done with doctors, and done with cancer.

It took time, but her hair grew back, she gained strength, and her laughter returned.

"I knew I could never go back to who I was," Wanda said. "The cancer journey had changed me. I kept thinking, *What was this all for?* I knew there was something that God wanted me to do. I just didn't know what."

Then, one morning, months after she had begun her recovery, she came across a very specific Bible verse: 2 Corinthians 1:4, "He comes alongside of us when we go through hard times, and before you know it, He brings us alongside someone else who is going through hard times so that we can be there for that person as God was there for us."

"God was speaking directly to me and giving me my charge," Wanda said. "I would unpack cancer, and cancer would become a big part of my life but in a different way."

Kneeling in prayer, Wanda sought God's direction, and suddenly she began to think of all the gifts of books and items of support that people had sent to encourage her during her treatment, including a basket filled with inspiration and love from her husband's family.

Suddenly, she knew what her mission was: to give support and encouragement to women and children diagnosed with cancer, in a basket. Each basket would be filled with books of encouragement, inspiration, and other helpful items that would support them through their journey.

It didn't take long for her Basket of Courage idea to get going.

What I thought would be two or three baskets a year turned into a hundred a year. We have since established Basket of Courage as a nonprofit organization and now send baskets all over the United States. Basket of Courage also provides a local Ronald McDonald House with fifty baskets annually for the kids that stay at the house during their illness.

Our prayer, for each basket, is for those whose faith has been shaken to be restored [in their faith] and for those searching to find hope and peace in Christ.

His love comforts; His grace sustains.

Sharing your story can be inspiring to others but also healing for you. The stories in this chapter are powerful examples of how people overcome devastating circumstance and not only survive but thrive. They each are amazing in their own way. If you have a personal story of hope, please share it at www.ShareYourStoryofHope.com. Help us continue to spread the message of hope.

Part II

BE EDUCATED: THE BIG IMPACT OF SMALL CHANGES

"An ounce of prevention
is worth a pound
of cure."

CHAPTER 3

GRANT YOURSELF IMMUNITY

C ancer is an epidemic. It takes our loved ones every day, and it respects no race, age, or gender. The word alone strikes immediate fear within us.

Cancer, according to the American Cancer Society, is the second leading cause of death in the United States, affecting one in three women and one in two men. There are more people every day who battle and defeat one type of cancer only to be diagnosed later in life with another form.

Have you ever wondered why?

Seventy years ago, the world rarely heard the word cancer. Store-bought foods processed with the litany of chemicals we see today did not exist at the turn of the twentieth century. Many of our great-grandparents cooked from scratch, used fresh fruits and vegetables from the garden, baked bread, and made meals with meat from animals raised on a farm. These foods weren't preserved with chemicals or injected with antibiotics or hormones. Preservatives, apart from age-old salt, were virtually unheard of.

Today, however, the standard American diet consists predominately of foods either processed or "enhanced" with chemicals.

In the past fifty years, synthetic chemicals have made their way into just about every industrial process and commercial product, with more than eighty thousand new chemicals invented since World War II.[5] They can be found in your cleaning products under the sink and in your medicine cabinet with your personal care products. They're in the air you breathe, the water you drink, and the food you eat.

Whether you want to be proactive about preventing a cancer diagnosis or rediagnosis, or, as a cancer patient, you're looking to preserve and support your immune system, then it's important to first understand the correlation between toxins entering your body and your immune system.

The Correlation between Cancer and the Immune System

The condition of your cells—your cellular health—is a measure of your health in general. When you're healthy on a cellular level, your immune system is healthy too. When toxins are loaded into your system through ingestion, inhala-

5 "Children and Toxic Chemicals," Mount Sinai Hospital, accessed May 10, 2016, http://www.mountsinai.org/patient-care/service-areas/children/areas-of-care/childrens-environmental-health-center/childrens-disease-and-the-environment/children-and-toxic-chemicals.

tion, or absorption, your body first has to get rid of them before it can do what it needs to do. This constant struggle creates a burden, ultimately weakening your immune system. By eliminating that chemical burden, your body is free to utilize the good things you put into it. Once it's free of synthetic chemicals, you can then boost your immune system with safe and healthy things such as an improved diet and good nutritional supplements.

Cancer often starts when your system becomes overloaded and your body can't keep up. The body can't fight off the burden, so it starts to mutate, leading to diseases, advanced aging, and cancer.

Free radical damage is also a source of cellular disruption. Although free radical damage occurs naturally in the body as part of the aging process, we drastically help that process along when we inhale pesticides in the air or put carcinogens such as formaldehyde on our skin. We speak more about free radical damage in chapter 5, but it's essential to understand that putting chemicals into our bodies can lead to damaging our bodies on a fundamental level.

Not all cancers, of course, have environmental origins. Some cancers are hereditary and no matter what you do to keep a clean and healthy lifestyle, that genetic tendency may still be triggered. But that hereditary risk should be an even bigger motivator to live in a healthier way and reduce any additional cancer risks.

The No Toxin Zone

The saying, "Necessity is the mother of invention," holds true in our own wellness journey. When we started our research, we realized how many other everyday consumers were as uninformed as we were about the common toxins that can be found all around us. As we began sharing ways to reduce the load on our immune systems, we discovered a real need to raise awareness. So we coauthored the No Toxin Zone, an educational awareness program focused on the three key functions through which toxins enter the body: inhalation, ingestion, and skin absorption. By understanding where you're under attack and the source of those attacks, you can grant yourself immunity from many toxins simply by refusing to allow them in your home or on your body.

In the first five years of sharing this program, more than thirty thousand people in our community became educated about the easy things that they could do to create a healthier environment and reduce their risk of developing cancer. When you consider the cancer statistics today, however, that number is a drop in the bucket. We want to reach *millions* with that message.

We believe prevention is foundational for all; those battling cancer as well as survivors need to be proactive about guarding their immune system.

There is a story of a philosophy professor who wanted to teach his class about being proactive when it comes to priorities in life. When the class began that day, he picked up a large, empty, mayonnaise jar and proceeded to fill it with rocks about two inches in diameter. Then he asked the students if the jar was full.

They agreed that it was full.

Then the professor picked up a box of pebbles and poured them into the jar. He shook the jar lightly, and the students watched as the pebbles rolled into the open areas between the rocks. The professor then again asked the students if the jar was full.

They chuckled and agreed that it was indeed full this time.

Once again, the professor put the jar down and added another item: sand. The tiny granules filled the last remaining open areas of the jar. He said to his students:

> Now I want you to recognize that this jar signifies your life. The rocks are the truly important things, such as family, health, and relationships. If all else was lost and only the rocks remained, your life would still be meaningful. The pebbles are the other things that matter in your life, such as work or school. The sand signifies the remaining "small stuff" and material possessions.
>
> If you put sand into the jar first, there is no room for the rocks or the pebbles. The same can be

applied to your lives. If you spend all your time and energy on the small stuff, you will never have room for the things that are truly important.

That lesson is one that we constantly strive to impart: pay attention to the things in life that are critical to your happiness and well-being. In the No Toxin Zone, the rocks that are foundational to our health are the decisions we make concerning what we breathe, what we ingest, and what goes on our skin. It is how we protect our immune system. The other important choices we make on our individual journey of wellness are the pebbles and sand.

Next we will take a deeper look at ingestion, inhalation, and skin absorption so that you can make better choices to strengthen your immune system and improve both your health and the health of your home. We believe that through simple changes and an increased awareness of the chemicals found in common products and their potential impacts on the human body, we can significantly reduce our exposure to toxins, strengthen our immune system, and create healthier homes.

Small Changes Make Big Impacts

Do you know your body's toxicity score?

1. How many processed foods (foods from a box or package) do you eat each day?
   a. one or less
   b. two to four servings
   c. five to nine servings
   d. ten or more servings

2. What type of cleaning products do you use?
   a. I am careful to use only green brands (naturally based ingredients).
   b. I use a combination of commercial and green brands.
   c. I use only commercial cleaning products (bleach, ammonia, disinfectants).

3. What type of personal care products (shampoo, lotion, skin care/cosmetics) do you use?
   a. I only use green brands (naturally based ingredients).
   b. I use some green brands.
   c. I don't use any green brands.

Visit BeWellAssured.com to complete our free, forty-five-second assessment and find out your body's toxicity score.

"You are what you eat. So don't be fast, cheap, easy or fake."

CHAPTER 4

YOU ARE WHAT YOU EAT

T

rue or false: you are what you eat. The answer is definitely true! Our health has everything to do with what we put in our bodies, but unfortunately, the standard American diet is heavy on calorie-dense foods. As a culture, we've become obsessed with instant gratification and convenience to the point where we don't even blink at the number of times in a week we visit our local fast-food chains.

At some point, the Western diet took a tragic turn and devalued what's most important to a healthy diet while pushing fatty foods to the forefront. Everything today is backward: processed foods reign supreme while fruits, vegetables, and whole grains are pushed aside. Cholesterol, salt, and sugars are loaded into our foods, and if that isn't bad enough, our general food consumption is critically short on dietary fiber, healthy fats, phytochemicals (plant-based nutrition), and many of the other nutrients that help protect our heart and our bodies and ward off cancer.

Processed, fake foods are constantly introduced to our bodies and, in turn, our bodies need to work extra hard to get rid of them. That increased workload takes energy away from other important functions, such as strengthening our immune system, and puts it into the detoxifying process, leaving us weaker and more vulnerable than we should be.

In his film *Doctored*, Jeff Hays discusses the sobering statistic that America only makes up 5 percent of the world's population, but it consumes 50 percent of the world's medications *and yet* remains one of the sickest countries on the planet. Why are we so sick? To find the answer, we need to look no further than the back of a cereal box—or any other boxed, canned, or artificially preserved food, for that matter.

The good news is that this situation is completely fixable! We as Americans have the resources and the choices to change these statistics. We are in complete control of what goes into our shopping carts, and with so many healthy eating options today, eating well can actually be fun and enjoyable. You may be just a few recipes away from lasting change!

The Sour Truth behind Sugar

Apart from chemicals, one of the biggest problems with processed foods is how much sugar they contain. Cancer thrives in a sugary environment, and too much sugar in the body can cause inflammatory messengers—cytokines—to spread and promote inflammation. While a little inflammation is good to help your body defend against foreign invaders, too much may actually help feed cancer cells and cause them to spread. Past epidemiological studies[6] have shown possible correlations between sugar, inflammation, and breast cancer development, and a study published in 2016 in *Cancer Research*[7] found a positive association between an increase in dietary sugar and the increased risk of breast cancer not only developing but also spreading.

Because of this, many cancer patients adopt ketogenic diets—ones that are low in carbs and high in fat—to starve off sugar in an attempt to treat cancer. But it's not easy! Sugar is addictive. Ingesting it causes a massive dopamine release in the brain, creating a high—a feeling of well-being that drives us to want more and more of it.

Sugar has no nutritional value. Along with its potential links to cancer and the spread of cancer, too much of it can overload the liver and lead to diabetes as well. But sugar can be sneaky, and it isn't always recognizable on a food label. On the next page are just a few of the names that sugar can go by.

---

6 "Sugar in Western Diets Increases Risk for Breast Cancer Tumors and Metastasis," University of Texas, MD Anderson Cancer Center, December 31, 2015, accessed May 10, 2016, https://www.mdanderson.org/newsroom/2015/12/sugar-in-western-diets.html.

7 Yan Jiang, Yong Pan, Patrea R. Rhea, Lin Tan, Mihai Gagea, Lorenzo Cohen, Susan M. Fischer, and Peiying Yang, "A Sucrose-Enriched Diet Promotes Tumorigenesis in Mammary Gland in Part through the 12-Lipoxygenase Pathway," Cancer Research 76, no. 1 (January 2016): 24–29, doi: 10.1158/0008-5472.CAN-14-3432.

SUGAR BY ANY OTHER NAME (FROM *WOMEN'S HEALTH* MAGAZINE)

agave nectar

barbados sugar

barley malt

beet sugar

blackstrap molasses

brown sugar

buttered syrup

cane juice crystals

cane sugar

caramel

carob syrup

castor sugar

confectioner's sugar

corn syrup

corn syrup solids

crystalline fructose

date sugar

demerara sugar

dextran

dextrose

diastatic malt

diatase

ethyl maltol

evaporated cane juice

Florida Crystals

fructose

fruit juice

fruit juice concentrate

galactose

glucose

glucose solids

golden sugar

golden syrup

grape sugar

high-fructose corn syrup

honey

icing sugar

invert sugar

lactose

malt syrup

maltodextrin

maltose

maple syrup

molasses

muscovado

organic raw sugar

panocha

raw sugar

refiner's syrup

rice syrup

sorghum syrup

sucrose

treacle

turbinado sugar

yellow sugar

A Second Chance for Sweet?

If all this makes you think twice about picking up that sugar packet, good! But don't reach for the little blue or pink sweeteners. The chemicals used to make sugar-free options such as aspartame and saccharin come with their own risks and connections to cancer.

In a letter to the FDA in 2003,[8] Mark Gold of the Aspartame Toxicity Information Center stated that the long-term ingestion of aspartame may cause or worsen a number of chronic illnesses, including brain tumors, epilepsy, Alzheimer's, lymphoma, and attention deficit disorder (ADD).

"We now have approximately 7,500 reports at an estimated reporting rate of 0.39%," wrote Gold. "This totals approximately 1.9 million *recognized* aspartame toxicity reactions in the US between 1982 and 1995. These reactions run anywhere from mild to very serious illnesses."

Additionally, Gold noted that "I would estimate that *at least* 7.6 million others are suffering from some symptoms related to aspartame use (many mild symptoms, but many serious ones as well) and do not recognize the connection."

Other sources state that since aspartame's release in the early 1980s, its ingestion has been associated with multiple allergenic, carcinogenic, metabolic, and neurotoxic effects,

8 "Reported Aspartame Toxicity Effects," Docket # 02P-0317, FDA Docket Submittals, January 12, 2002, accessed May 10, 2016, http://www.fda.gov/ohrms/dockets/dailys/03/jan03/012203/02p-0317_emc-000199.txt.

including the erosion of intelligence and short-term memory. A short list of health problems that may be associated with aspartame ingestion includes:

- brain tumors and brain cancer
- leukemia and lymphoma
- birth defects
- diabetes
- multiple sclerosis
- Parkinson's disease
- arthritis
- chronic fatigue syndrome
- epilepsy/seizures
- migraines
- heart disease
- weight gain

There are some safer alternatives out there, such as stevia, sucralose, and xylitol, but these options are still being debated.

In the end, the answer always comes back to this: whole, unprocessed, natural foods are the best.

Unexpected Chemicals

True or false: You should only shop organic.

False! It's a great idea to shop organic when at all possible, based on availability and budget, but not all fruits and vegetables are equal when it comes to the danger of absorbing pesticides, which is the main reason for buying organic.

Why are some types of produce more prone to absorbing pesticides than others? In most cases, this risk is determined by how well the fruit or vegetable is protected by its outer layer. Those with a thick protective layer of skin, such as pineapples, are less risky than strawberries or other berries. However, we also need to be aware that plant roots absorb substances from the soil, including herbicides and other toxins that settle there over time. Organically grown plants have much less of a risk of this. So pineapples grown in toxic soil, even though they have a thick protective layer of skin, will absorb that toxin.

A 2010 report issued by the President's Cancer Panel recommends eating produce without pesticides to reduce your risk of getting cancer and other diseases.

According to the Environmental Working Group—an organization of scientists, researchers, and policy makers— eating certain types of chemical-free organic produce can reduce the amount of toxins you consume on a daily basis by as much as 80 percent.[9] The group released two lists to help consumers understand which types of produce are best purchased as organically grown products and which ones don't necessarily have to be. They call these lists the "Dirty Dozen" and the "Clean 15." These lists are compiled and updated yearly using data from the US Department of Agri-

9 "Clean Fifteen," Environmental Working Group (EWG), accessed May 10, 2016, http://www.ewg.org/foodnews/clean_fifteen_list.php.

culture on the amount of pesticide residue found in nonorganic fruits and vegetables after they had been washed. You can check out the full list at www.foodnews.org.

"The Clean 15"

These are the fruits and veggies that the EWG states are generally safe to eat when grown conventionally:

asparagus	eggplants	mangoes
avocados	frozen sweet peas	onions
cabbage	grapefruit	papayas
cantaloupe	honeydew melon	pineapple
cauliflower	kiwi	sweet corn

"The Dirty Dozen"

On the other hand, you should buy the organically grown variety of the following fruits and veggies, whenever possible, due to their tendency to absorb any pesticides, fungicides, and other chemicals sprayed on them during the growing process:

apples	cucumbers	spinach
celery	grapes	strawberries
cherries	nectarines	sweet bell peppers
cherry tomatoes	peaches	tomatoes

In general, the thinner the membrane of the fruit or vegetable, the more consideration you should give to purchasing the organically grown variety of that produce.

Fruits and veggies are not the only foods in which harmful chemicals may be hiding. Take dairy products and milk, for example. The hormones injected into dairy cows and into calves to fatten them into harvestable hamburger as quickly as possible have been found to affect children at young ages. In some circles there is a debate about whether early menstruation can be linked to these genetically modified hormones found in meats and dairy products.[10]

Additionally, meats loaded with hormones and antibiotics also send low doses of antibiotics into the body, making it harder for antibiotics to do their job when they're really needed.

When it comes to meat and dairy, it's wise to be thoughtful about using organic versions whenever possible. Pasture-raised chicken and eggs are a good choice since more natural diets lead to more natural products. So your pasture-raised cheeses, butters, and meats are always going to be better alternatives.

Lastly, the value of looking at labels cannot be understated, and that applies not only to what goes into your body permanently but also temporarily. Take toothpaste, for example. It may only be in your mouth for a couple minutes, but a little of it always finds a way down the back of your throat. Shockingly, many toothpastes—even ones approved

10 Joel Fuhrman, MD, "Girls' Early Puberty: What Causes It, and How to Avoid "*Huffington Post* blog, updated July 6, 2011, http://www.huffingtonpost.com/joel-fuhrman-md/girls-early-puberty_b_857167.html.

by the American Dental Association (ADA)—contain sugar substitutes such as saccharin and other artificial flavoring agents. In these cases, finding a toothpaste with a sweetener such as xylitol can help you fight tooth decay without worrying over ingesting potential carcinogens.

The Dirt on Vitamins

If we are what we eat, how can we make sure we're really protecting our bodies from disease? In short, one of the best things we can do for our health is make sure we're getting the proper amount of vitamins and minerals every day. In fact, the *Journal of American Medicine* (JAMA) published a study in 2002 stating that "inadequate intake of several vitamins is associated with chronic disease."[11] But why, in a developed country, would we lack the fruits, vegetables, and proteins we need to naturally keep our vitamin intake at its optimal level? The answer may be closer than we think.

Our soil today has had far more demand of it than ever before. As a result, it has become very nutrient deficient, and the use of pesticides in our farm fields has caused some ripples in the pond.

For instance, one orange today has about eight times less nutritional value than an orange grown fifty years ago.[12]

11 Fairfield K. M., and R. H. Fletcher, "Vitamins for Chronic Disease Prevention in Adults: Scientific Review," *JAMA* 287, no. 23 (2002): 3116–3126, doi:10.1001/jama.287.23.3116.
12 "Do Fruits and Veggies Have Enough Nutrients Today?" Healthy You Naturally, accessed May 10, 2016, http://www.healthyyounaturally.com/

Many fields are no longer kept on a rotation that allows old crops to decompose back into the earth, which means the soil isn't being replenished naturally. And as land supply dwindles and food demand increases, we continue to put more stress on the soil available, which means that, with each unreplenished crop growth, the vitamin and mineral supply diminishes even more.

The Secret in the Supplement

To balance out this deficiency, we need to supplement our diet with vitamins and minerals, but before you grab the first bottle of multivitamins off the shelf, one important element you should look for is how well those vitamins are going to be absorbed by your body.

Many people would be shocked to find that several of the top advertised supplements provide less than 10 percent of absorption into the body. With poor delivery systems, not only do very little of those vitamins actually work their way into your system but they also throw off free radicals, which are linked to a variety of diseases, cell breakdown, and aging.

Free radicals occur when weak bonds between two molecules split, leaving one molecule with an odd number of electrons, causing it to become unstable. When that occurs, the newly formed free radical tends to grab the closest electron to it, rendering another molecule unstable

edu/fruits-veggies-enough-nutrients.htm.

and starting a chain reaction. If the reaction continues, it may result in damaging a living cell.

So how do we fight free radicals? With antioxidants! When free radicals are running rampant, antioxidants provide an extra electron for free radicals to latch onto. Since antioxidants are stable even when they lose an electron, they stop the process of molecular instability, thus helping to prevent cellular damage.

Free radicals occur naturally in the process of metabolism, and they can be helpful to our immune system when they're used to render invading viruses and bacteria neutral, but they can also grow at excessive rates when triggered by negative environmental factors such as pesticides and pollution. And because free radical damage builds up over time and with age, our bodies become more susceptible to damage.

A good multivitamin supplement is designed to survive the acidic environment of the stomach and get into the body's cells with a high rate of absorption. This is important because vitamins and minerals need to pass through the stomach and into the small intestine to be absorbed into the body. Because there is a difference between the pH in the stomach and in the small intestine, minerals can crystallize, which prevents them from reaching the bloodstream. They will be eliminated from the body without delivering any benefits.

So looking for a supplement with a proper binding process that allows all those important nutrients to get to your cells and doesn't cause free radical damage is important, especially if you're not getting what you need from your daily diet. You wouldn't want to take a vitamin supplement if it's only going to cause more harm than good. In looking into your current supplement's absorption rates, if the binding process isn't apparent on the label, it is a good idea to do your research to find out what the absorption rate is.

Take a Load Off: Gut Health and Probiotics

Speaking of the stomach, we are learning more every day that the gut is almost as much a control center of the body as the brain, which means we need to keep it clean and healthy. Fiber, digestive enzymes, fermented foods, and drinks, as well as a good probiotic will definitely help with this, as a healthy gut is a major contributor to a healthy immune system.

Probiotics are essentially a dense collection of beneficial bacteria that helps maintain balance in the gut. These bacteria support your immune system, break down food for digestion, support the absorption of nutrients, help with eliminating toxins, and reinforces good bacteria to keep bad bacteria at a minimum. Ideally, a healthy human gut contains 85 percent of beneficial and 15 percent of bad bacteria. When a strong balance like this is maintained, your gut flora can help protect you from more than a hundred different diseases and health problems, including celiac disease, irritable bowel syndrome, metabolic syndrome, diabetes, Epstein-Barr virus, acne, herpes, chronic fatigue syndrome, liver disease, food and wheat allergies, and a number of other ailments.[13] When choosing a probiotic, the best ones will likely provide the following information:

CFU/ml	This is the number of colony-forming units, or living organisms, in a single dose. More is better, so if you're trying to decide between one with eight billion CFU/ml and one with ten billion CFU/ml, it's probably better to go for the latter.
Genus and species of bacteria	Some of the best probiotics contain one or more of the following strains: ,lactobacillus, streptococcus thermophiles, saccharomyces boulardii, bacillus coagulans, and bifidobacteria.
Storage tips	Living probiotics do best when kept in dark, cool environments. Proper storage information should be included to prevent unwanted bacterial growth and to keep your probiotics healthy after the seal is broken.
Expiration date	Because probiotics are living bacteria, an expiration date should clearly be stated on the packaging and adhered to by the user.

Remember, maintaining a healthy gut is important for preventing and healing many ailments. If you want proper nutrient uptake, protection against viruses and pathogens,

13 "Probiotics," GreenMedInfo, accessed May 10, 2016, http://www.green-medinfo.com/substance/probiotics?ed=5161

proper metabolism, and weight regulation, as well as good nutrient creation, keep your gut full of good flora with proper probiotics.

Pharmaceuticals

True or false: Pharmaceuticals are the only solution to treating illness.

False! There are times that lifesaving medications need to be available to us. The problem we run into is that, oftentimes, the "pill plan" is given as our only option. However, there are often a number of natural alternatives that may be just as effective. Chronic issues such as type 2 diabetes, depression, and heart health can greatly benefit from lifestyle changes including choosing to eat healthy food and natural supplements. In some cases, these changes can lead people to reduce or even eliminate the need for medications.

Unfortunately, the theme of Western medicine is very much cause and effect: manage the symptoms but rarely go after the root cause. Instead, if a person is diagnosed with type 2 diabetes, for instance, doctors might just hand him or her a pill to manage it. Or if patients have high blood pressure, their doctors may prescribe a medication regimen to bring it back down.

But some people don't want to manage symptoms. They want to get to the root cause and find a cure. We applaud those people. Those are the "be the change" people that are joining today's wellness movement.

Three Natural Living Testimonials

DEPRESSION

Penny saw the benefits of clean eating, organic shopping, and proper supplementation firsthand when she decided that she was sick of dealing with the side effects of medications and wanted to overcome her depression and anxiety naturally. Over the course of a year, she went through some gut detoxification, began natural supplementation, and focused on eating a more organic diet. Today she's off all of her medications, and she's lost fifty pounds. Her anxiety has disappeared and, overall, she feels much better.

CHILDHOOD ADHD

Imbalances in the body and excesses of processed food and sugars in the diet can lead to some unexpected side effects. Recently, Melinda was having trouble with her son's behavior at school. He was having trouble focusing and was frequently reprimanded by his teachers. Instead of immediately putting him on medication for ADD or ADHD, she first removed processed foods and a lot of the sugar from his diet and began supplementing with omega-3s. His teachers quickly noticed a big improvement in his school behavior, focus, and cognition and inquired whether his mom had made any changes. They were amazed that these changes were not medication related.

CHOLESTEROL

At age twenty-three, Paul was diagnosed with high cholesterol. His LDL cholesterol level was ranging in the 300s; a healthy level is considered to be 100 mg/dL or below. For more than a decade he went on and off statin drugs in an attempt to lower that number, until one day, in his midthirties, he found out about phytosterols as a natural alternative for reducing cholesterol.

Within ninety days of starting on phytosterols, his cholesterol level went down to the 150s with absolutely no medication, just the natural supplements and positive changes to his diet. It was pretty dramatic. And even though his condition is hereditary, those natural changes spoke powerfully to the benefits of healthy living and proper supplementation.

Melinda and Paul can testify, as Penny did, that our body has the amazing ability to heal itself. Eating healthy food and getting necessary vitamins and nutrients are essential. Even if these changes don't lead to reducing or eliminating your need to take medications, natural, whole foods are simply better for your body and help support a healthy immune system.

Cleaning House, Gradually

Moving to a completely clean, healthy, organic food diet is not an easy process, especially if you are used to a diet that relies heavily on processed foods, as many Americans are. But just dropping your old lifestyle and immediately switching

100 percent to a new one can be a recipe for failure. For a change that you want to last a lifetime instead of a weekend, approach it gradually.

One of these functional, enforceable approaches is the *80/20 rule.*

When trying to make healthy eating changes, work toward changing your diet so that 80 percent of what you eat is clean, whole, and healthy, while leaving 20 percent that is not.

It would be great to live a completely clean, 100 percent healthy lifestyle, but it takes commitment. So, in reality, if we can do 80 percent clean and 20 percent not clean, then our bodies and our immune systems will fare much better than they otherwise would have done.

The Add-In Rule

Instead of the "taking away" and depravation usually tied to changes in diet, the add-in rule focuses instead on the positives. For example, by adding eight glasses of water a day to your diet the water fills you up so that you don't have room for, say, three glasses of soda that day. By focusing on adding in the good, the bad automatically starts to weed itself out.

Neither of these approaches to changing your diet need to be done overnight—nor should they. To make a lasting change, it always helps to work toward your goal gradually, allowing yourself time to shed old habits and shake old cravings.

With the add-in rule, for example, start by adding only two glasses of water a day for a week and then up the glasses to three or four the following week.

You don't have to go from nothing to everything all at once. Gradual change leads to lasting change and sets you up for success.

Small Changes Make Big Impacts

- *Keep a food diary:* For one week, write down everything you eat. Circle any of the foods that are considered clean. How close are you to the 80/20 rule? This will help you gauge where to add in healthier options.

- *Meal planning:* Plan one week of meals, and then create a grocery list. Circle the items that are on the "Dirty Dozen" list, and substitute those with an organic version. Which whole foods can you substitute for processed ones?

"Environmental pollution is an incurable disease. It can only be prevented."

BARRY COMMONER

CHAPTER 5

LET'S CLEAR THE AIR

N ow let's really clear the air. We breathe in and exhale about ten thousand quarts of air each day. That's close to 2,500 gallons of air! So it's safe to say that clean air is not only important to our health, but it's also one of the fastest ways for airborne toxins to enter our bodies.

Airborne toxins—both hidden and not so hidden— affect our health every day. The obvious ones, of course, are pollution, cigarette smoke, carbon monoxide, and pesticides. But what about the toxins that we spray in our homes every day, such as bleach and ammonia, or the ones that are released through the off-gassing of products such as fresh paint and chemically treated wood? What about the pesticides found in common disinfectants?

According to the National Resources Defense Council,[14] More than *eighty thousand chemicals* available in the United

14 "Toxic Chemicals," National Resources Defense Council, accessed May 10, 2016, http://www.nrdc.org/health/toxics.asp.

States have *never been fully tested for their toxic effects* on our health and environment, and toxic chemical exposure has been associated with many health risks, including cancer.

Unfortunately, laws such as the Toxic Substances Control Act (TSCA) of 1976 have done little to prevent the use of dangerous chemicals in everyday products. The weaknesses in the TSCA have allowed chemical companies to delay regulations and final health assessments by the Environmental Protection Agency, sometimes for decades, with the result that most chemicals are "innocent until proven guilty."

And yet, the law, now more than forty years old, remains unchanged. Today, common household products can contain any number of chemicals with no proven safety record.

Consider the warning label language on a bottle of common household tile cleaner:

> WARNING: Causes substantial but temporary eye injury and can irritate skin. For sensitive skin or prolonged use, wear gloves. Do not get in eyes or on clothing. Vapors may irritate. Use only in well-ventilated areas. Avoid prolonged breathing of vapors. **Not recommended for use by persons with heart conditions or chronic respiratory problems such as asthma, emphysema, or obstructive lung disease.** Due to irritating nature, may be harmful if swallowed. FIRST AID: IF IN EYES: Hold eye open and rinse slowly and gently with water for 15–20 minutes. Remove contact lenses, if present, after the first

5 minutes, then continue rinsing eyes. IF ON SKIN OR CLOTHING: Take off contaminated clothing. Rinse skin immediately with plenty of water for 15–20 minutes. IF INHALED: Move person to fresh air. If the person is not breathing, call 911 or ambulance, then give artificial respiration, preferably mouth-to-mouth, if possible. IF SWALLOWED: Call a poison control center or doctor for treatment advice. Have person sip a glassful of water if able to swallow. Do not induce vomiting unless told to do so by a poison control center or doctor. Do not give anything by mouth to an unconscious person. Call a poison control center or doctor for further treatment advice. Have the product container or label with you when calling a poison control center or doctor or going for treatment. PHYSICAL AND CHEMICAL HAZARDS: **This product contains bleach. Do not use or mix this product with other household chemicals such as products containing ammonia, toilet bowl cleaners, rust removers, vinegar, or acid.** To do so will release hazardous gases.

How often do we take the time to really read the warning labels on the backs of our cleaning products? How often do we take the time to dig up a pair of kitchen gloves to wear before spraying down a countertop? If we do get it on our skin, do we really take fifteen to twenty minutes to rinse it off?

Many consumers use products like this everyday with the utmost trust that no company would sell us a product that could harm or even kill us. But one look at those warning labels tells a different tale.

Carrie's Story

The mother of four children, three of whom were elementary school-age, Carrie also had a toddler who was born a preemie. The little girl had all kinds of respiratory issues that required the constant use of oxygen as well as albuterol treatments multiple times a day.

Because her daughter's immune system was also at risk, Carrie had an automatic disinfecting spray in her house that went off every fifteen minutes, and she wiped down everything with bleach wipes, to the point where she would just pour the liquid from an empty wipe container onto tables and countertops to clean them off. Everything her daughter touched was wiped with bleach, from her high chair to the windowpanes that she frequently pressed her little nose and lips against.

What Carrie wasn't aware of was that all-too-important information found on the warning label of any product containing bleach, including the previously shown warning label. Bleach aggravates the respiratory system and is especially harmful to people suffering from respiratory conditions.

At first, she was shocked when she found this out and then angry. Here she was trying to do everything she could to help her daughter, trying to be a good mom by reducing the amount of germs so her daughter could be healthy, and the whole time, the products she thought were helping were, instead, taxing her little girl's already-fragile immune system.

Carrie immediately got rid of all the bleach in her house, got rid of the automatic disinfecting spray, opened her windows, and detoxified her house. Today her daughter no longer needs oxygen, and it only took a couple months after Carrie cleared the air for her daughter to come off of the albuterol treatments. Since then, she hasn't needed to go to the hospital once for respiratory issues.

Sadly, Carrie's story is a common one. Most of us think all these chemicals are making our homes safe and healthy when, in reality, they may be contributing to health issues.

Formaldehyde Stinks

Another unnerving example of a common household toxin is formaldehyde. We talk more about this dangerous carcinogen in the next chapter because of its presence as a preservative in products that we apply directly to our skin but also because it's an airborne danger. Any length of airborne exposure to formaldehyde can result in irritations to the eye, nose, and throat and cause symptoms of respiratory illness.

So why are we introducing it into our homes? Today we build our homes to be energy efficient, to keep air in and prevent excessive use of our air conditioners and heaters. But in keeping all that air in, we keep the fresh air out, leaving the airborne chemicals in our homes with no way out. According to the EPA, "Indoor air levels of many pollutants may be 2–5 times, and occasionally, more than 100 times higher than outdoor levels. Indoor air pollutants are of particular concern because most people spend as much as 90% of their time indoors."[15]

For this very reason, it's been debated that women who stay at home rather than working outside the home are at a greater risk for cancer.

In 2014 the National Academy of Sciences released an assessment of formaldehyde[16] as a follow-up to the National Toxicology Program's Twelfth Report on Carcinogens, in which formaldehyde was recommended for listing as "known to be a human carcinogen." The assessment completely agreed with this finding, noting that there is sufficient evidence that formaldehyde is the cause of at least two types of upper respiratory tract cancer, as well as myeloid leukemia.

The good news is this is something we can avoid. Opening our homes up to fresh air, eliminating products that

---

15 "Basic Information: Air and Radiation," Environmental Protection Agency, last modified February 23, 2016, https://www3.epa.gov/air/basic.html.

16 "Review of the Formaldehyde Assessment in the National Toxicology Program 12th Report on Carcinogens," Board on Environmental Studies and Toxicology, National Academy of Sciences, August 2014, accessed May 10, 2016, http://dels.nas.edu/resources/static-assets/materials-based-on-reports/reports-in-brief/formaldehyde-report-highlights-Final2.pdf.

contain formaldehyde, and being educated on what is safe to use are ways to be proactive in our health.

Bleach: The Killer in Our Cupboards

The number-one killer in our cupboards is bleach. Bleach has a rare ability to change forms. It's a major asthma trigger because it aggravates the lower membranes of the respiratory tract, causing wheezing and coughing. Yet, television commercials market bleach as though it's a safe cleaner. Have you noticed how many of the commercials feature moms holding chemical-soaked wipes or sponges without a glove in sight? They are wiping down high chair trays and countertops where food is prepared with that big, sparkling, "I'm-killing-germs" grin, but the truth is that they are unleashing a host of toxins with every spray.

Compare that to the Occupational Safety and Health Administration (OSHA) information sheet, *Protecting Workers Who Use Cleaning Chemicals*, which, among other things, requires giving workers training on "personal protective equipment required for using the cleaning product, such as gloves, safety goggles, and respirators."

Cleaning product commercials create a false sense of safety, particularly when you consider some of the warnings on the back of standard household cleaners such as bleach:

DANGER: For prolonged use wear gloves. Wash hands after contact. Avoid breathing vapors. Use in well ventilated areas. KEEP OUT OF REACH OF CHILDREN.

May cause severe irritation or damage to eyes and skin. Harmful if swallowed; nausea, vomiting, and burning sensation of the mouth and throat may occur. The following medical conditions may be aggravated by exposure to high concentrations of vapor or mist: heart conditions, or chronic respiratory problems such as asthma, chronic bronchitis or obstructive lung disease. Some clinical reports suggest a low potential for skin sensitization upon exaggerated exposure to sodium hypochlorite, particularly on damaged or irritated skin.

Most people don't realize how many products out there contain bleach. Toilet bowl cleaners, dishwasher detergents, and tile cleaners are just a few examples, and many times, they are used concurrently with, or sprayed in the same area as, a product containing ammonia, such as window cleaner. This mixing of chlorine bleach and an acid such as ammonia (or vinegar) can create chlorine gas, which at low levels can cause breathing problems and at high levels can cause chest pain, fluid in the lungs, and even death. If the gas mixes with water, it can create hydrochloric acid, which can cause burns when touched or inhaled.[17]

---

17 "Common Cleaning Products May Be Dangerous When Mixed," New Jersey Department of Health and Senior Services, Consumer and Environ-

Ammonia Alternative

Most window cleaners are nothing but the toxic chemical ammonia mixed with water and a little blue, green, or yellow dye. Inhaling ammonia can cause all kinds of damage, from throat and nose irritation to airway destruction and respiratory failure, and skin exposure can lead to chemical burns.

Instead of keeping a dangerous poison like this around just to keep the windows sparkly, consider mixing up a bottle of equal portions of distilled white vinegar and water and wiping down the surface with crumpled newspaper or a paper towel for a gorgeous shine.

Pesticides Undercover

Another little known fact is that cleaners with the term *disinfectant* on the label contain a registered pesticide, the chemical that is actually killing the germs.

By definition, a pesticide is "a chemical preparation for destroying plant, fungal, or animal pests." Most of us hear the term *pesticide* and think about weed killers and commercially grown crops. But many of us are unaware that the

mental Services, accessed May 10, 2016, http://www.state.nj.us/health/eoh/cehsweb/bleach_fs.pdf.

majority of our exposure to pesticides occurs right in our own homes. These pesticides are known carcinogens, and yet we are spraying them liberally and inhaling them, practically on a daily basis.

Overspray too is a common concern that few of us consider. Think about it. Every day we spray cleaners on surfaces, but not all of that liquid is going to the same spot. Overspray can hit the floor, walls, carpets, and even food, without our noticing, leaving the liquid to be absorbed into the skin of a bare foot, a crawling baby's hands, or the footpads of a dog or cat. It's just one more reason for us to really pay attention to what we are spraying around our homes every day.

To list all of the common names for pesticides would probably take a whole other book, but if you're interested, you can find out more at the EPA's pesticide registration site found at www.EPA.gov.

Becoming aware of what we are using to clean our homes every day is easy. Get under your cabinets, and start reading labels. Do a little research and start ditching those products that are harming you and your family with every breath.

Give BPA the Boot

BPA, or bisphenol-A, is a hormone disruptor that can be found in the vast majority of plastic containers, from insulated travel mugs to water bottles and even canned goods, as many metal

cans are lined on the interior with an anticorrosive plastic.

The ideal solution is to use glass containers, but if that's just not practical, look for BPA-free plastics. Coffee k-cups that are not clearly labeled BPA-free also need to be given the boot, as they release harmful toxins into your coffee upon brewing.

What a Gas

We mentioned outgassing when it comes to formaldehyde and building materials, but that's not the only product passively emitting fumes in the home—not by far. Outgassing, or offgassing, is the process in which a solid releases a gas. Think about the last time you walked down the cleaning supply aisle in your local grocery store or picked up your dry cleaning. What did you smell? Fumes, fragrances, vapors—all artificial, all trying to entice you with the scent of "clean" while, in fact, releasing any number of harmful chemicals into the air. In fact, one of the most commonly recognized outgassing scents comes from that distinctive "new" smell associated with many consumer goods.

Here are some helpful tips: Launder clothes whenever possible versus dry-cleaning. When you do need to have clothes dry-cleaned, make sure you remove them from the bag, put them in a room that you can open windows, and air them out. Whenever you install new carpeting or you buy new furniture, open the windows to clear the air, and let the chemicals in those fabrics and fibers escape.

Small Changes Make Big Impacts

CABINET CHECK

When was the last time you looked at the ingredient list and/or warning labels on the common products found around your home? The following items are often found to contain toxins that can harm your health every day:

air fresheners	carpet
disinfectants	laundry detergents
drain cleaners	bleach
oven cleaners	stain removers
window cleaners	fabric softeners
floor/furniture polish	shampoos
spot removers	dandruff shampoos
all-purpose cleaners	deodorants
toilet bowl cleaners	mousse and hair sprays
chlorinated scouring	mouthwash
powders	breath sprays
dishwasher detergents	perfume/cologne
dishwashing liquids	cosmetics
carpet shampoos	

As always, it's important to do your own research. Find manufacturing companies that have safe ingredients. The more we support these companies, the more we help create change. Small changes truly do make a big impact!

"Take care of your body. It's the only place you have to live."

CHAPTER 6

PORE HEALTH?

A re you in pore health? Think about it: your skin is your largest organ, but do you really know what you're putting on it?

Skin absorption is the second fastest way in which toxins enter the immune system—inhalation being the fastest—and yet the products we put on our skin and the cleaners we touch every day are far less regulated than the food we eat and the medicines we take. But why? Don't we realize how much of a sponge our skin is for everything we put on it?

Doctors, for example, use patch technology to treat all kinds of issues, from its most well known use as a smoking cessation tool to boosting hormone levels, providing transdermal contraception options, and facilitating pain management. In fact, at the time of this writing there are more than one hundred drugs that are administered via skin application[18] including creams and ointments and nineteen drug or

---

18 Prausnitz, M. R., and R. Langer, "Transdermal Drug Delivery," Nature Biotechnology 26, no. 11: 1261–1268, http://doi.org/10.1038/nbt.1504.

drug combinations approved by the Food and Drug Administration (FDA) to be administered using a patch.

The Lavender Test

If you are curious about how quickly and thoroughly your skin absorbs what is applied to it, take a small drop of lavender essential oil, dab it on your wrist, and wait a few minutes. In most cases, you should find that you get a warm, sweet, almost licorice-like taste in the back of your throat. That's the lavender! And that's a simple example of how quickly products can permeate your skin and travel through your blood stream.

With so much evidence about the amazing absorption qualities of our skin, it can only benefit you to take a few minutes and explore exactly what we are putting on it. What you find out may be shocking.

A Word from Jen: Getting Rid of Hormone Disruptors

For six years, my husband and I tried to have kids. I never even thought about toxins, and if I heard the word *pesticide*, I thought about fertilizer or bug killers. I never considered that toxins might have something to do with our difficulty in conceiving.

In 2001, we adopted our first baby. Then, in 2002, we did in vitro, and I became pregnant with twins. We were so excited! The in vitro process was difficult, and my inability to conceive naturally was still unexplained.

In 2004, I came across information about toxins I was completely unaware of, such as the effect that chemicals in personal care and cleaning products could have on my children's health. Having a two-year-old and one-year-old twins motivated me to start shopping for safer products. Two months after I switched out our family's personal care and cleaning products, as well as my own cosmetic line, we were surprisingly pregnant with our fourth child.

It was a huge shock. Just these few changes, made in the course of only two months, had allowed my body to conceive naturally. As I researched more, I discovered that there are seven different cleaners that have been linked to reproductive disorders and that hormone disruptors can be found in many skin care products and cosmetics.

This unexpected pregnancy became the catalyst for me to begin telling others the truth about toxins.

A Word from Kim: Banishing Eczema

For about twenty-five years, I had chronic eczema. It was awful: cracked, bleeding skin, sleeping with gloves on my hand every night, and slathering every type of prescription and over-the-counter goop I could find on the rashes—to no effect. I saw dermatologists and used steroid creams, but nothing got rid of it.

Then I started to do some research, and as Jen had done, I too switched out my cosmetics, skin care, personal care, and household cleaning products. As a result, I've been eczema-free for more than a decade.

The same thing happened with my daughter and Jen's sister-in-law. A week after I changed my daughter's products, her eczema was gone. Jen's sister-in-law's psoriasis cleared up after three weeks. She was able to wear makeup to work for the first time in eight years.

What Goes into Your Skin

We know the following pages contain a lot of technical content and some chemical names. Although it is a lot of information, it is good to be aware of when doing your own product research.

In 1989 the National Institute of Occupational Safety and Health (NIOSH) analyzed 2,983 chemicals used in personal and cosmetic products, as well as home care products, and found that

- 884 of these chemicals were toxic,
- 774 caused acute toxicity,
- 146 caused tumors,
- 218 caused reproductive complications,

- 314 caused biological mutation, and
- 376 caused skin and eye irritations.

Another study, released in 1990 and conducted by the Toronto Indoor Air Conference over a period of fifteen years, found that women who worked in the home were 54 percent more likely to die from cancer than those who worked in other environments, due to their increased exposure to household chemicals.[19]

When we don't see the damage actually happening, it's hard to realize the toll these chemicals are taking on our bodies. We can't see our cellular health. We can see diseases, or symptoms of diseases, telling us that something isn't right, but we can't see the destruction taking place when we handle a disinfectant wipe with bare hands or take a deep whiff of bleach.

The body is designed with the capacity to heal itself. Think about when you cut your finger. You don't have to tell your body to heal the wound and create a scab. It already knows to do that. It is an incredible machine with an intricate balance of systematic inner workings, but just because the effect of chemicals isn't evident now or five years from now, that doesn't mean they are not having a long-term effect on your health. The chemicals coming in contact with your skin are taxing your immune system with every application.

---

19 Michael DeJong, "The Dirty Word in Clean," *Huffington Post* blog, May 25, 2011, http://www.huffingtonpost.com/michael-dejong/the-dirty-word-in-clean_b_171464.html.

The Chemical Culprits

We could spend the rest of this book discussing all of the chemicals out there that are potentially harmful, but it's far easier to use great resources such as SaferCosmetics.org to help you look up the comparative safety of different skin and personal care products.

We do however want to cover the four chemical culprits that we feel are most important to avoid, starting with formaldehyde.

Formaldehyde

Formaldehyde is a preservative that many companies use because it is inexpensive. It's a colorless, poisonous gas that is used to make everything from disinfectants to building materials to personal care products and even cigarettes. The EPA also considers formaldehyde to be a possible carcinogen, which means there's a chance that it causes cancer.

This is definitely something to avoid, right? And all you have to do is look for it on product labels. If "formaldehyde" is listed on the ingredient list, don't buy it.

Unfortunately, it's not that easy. As do so many other potentially dangerous products in the world, this one goes by many names, including:

formalin	hcho
Formol*	BFV*
oxomethane	methylene glycol
methanal	paraform
Fyde*	Fannoform*
formalin 40	methanediol
methyl aldehyde	Lysoform*
Karsan*	morbicid
methylene oxide	polyoxmethylene
methaldehyde	superlysoform
formic aldehyde	*denotes trade name
oxymethylene	
Formalith*	

Instead of containing formaldehyde, many skin, body, hair, and hygiene products contain formaldehyde releasers. These chemicals, popularly used as preservatives and antimicrobials, are designed to decompose as slowly as possible in order to have a longer-lasting preservative effect, but as they break down, they release formaldehyde.

Not only does this mean that the awful, scented hand lotion that Aunt Gladys sent you many moons ago, still sitting unused in the linen closet, is likely releasing formaldehyde into your home, but there's also a risk that these chemicals are releasing formaldehyde even after they've been absorbed into the body.

Once again, formaldehyde releasers go by many names. Several of the more popular ones include:

- quaternium-15
- imidazolidinyl urea

- benzylhemiformal
- DMDM hydantoin
- sodium hydroxymethylglycinate
- diazolindinyl urea

Time to Change the Sheets

If your bed sheets are labeled "permanent press" or are a polyester/cotton blend, chances are that they are also coated in a formaldehyde-releasing resin. If you've been having respiratory trouble, watery eyes, or bouts of insomnia at night, consider changing your sheets to untreated, all-cotton ones, particularly ones without that "no-iron" label.

Triclosan

Triclosan is an antimicrobial agent that can be found in a variety of products, from toothpaste to deodorant to soap. It was first developed for doctors as a surgical scrub, but because it was found to kill bacteria and fungus so well, it's been added to a number of items in need of fungus-fighting capabilities—from shoes to shaving products.

The problem, however, is that triclosan has been linked to hormone disruption as well as antibiotic resistance, and it's one of those chemicals that stays in the body for undeter-mined lengths of time.[20]

Concerns continue to come up regarding its use, par-ticularly its potential associations with endocrine disruption and bioaccumulation.

OTHER NAMES FOR TRICLOSAN

- triclocarban

Phthalates (pronounced, thal-āt)

Phthalates are a group of chemicals most commonly used to make plastics stronger, yet more flexible, but manufacturers have also found a use for them in cosmetics. Phthalates are added to nail polish to make it stronger and less brittle, to hair sprays to make them more flexible, and to cosmetics and soaps to fix fragrances.

Phthalates have been linked to endocrine disruption, cancer, and developmental toxicity and have been banned from use in cosmetics in the European Union.[21] In the United States phthalate diethylphthalate (DEP) is still found in a variety of cosmetics.

---

20 "Chemicals of Concern," Campaign for Safe Cosmetics, 2016, http://www.safecosmetics.org/get-the-facts/chemicals-of-concern/.

21 Ibid.

OTHER NAMES FOR PHTHALATES

- dibutylphthalate (DBP)
- dimethylphthalate (DMP)
- diethylphthalate (DEP)
- bis(2-ethylhexyl) phthalate (DEHP)

Parabens

Parabens are a common preservative in cosmetics and are also used to prevent the growth of several types of microorganisms. They're also considered by some to be an endocrine disruptor, acting in a way that is similar to estrogen in the body, and they are associated with certain forms of breast cancer.

OTHER NAMES FOR PARABENS

- ethylparaben
- butylparaben
- isobutylparaben
- isopropylparaben
- methylparaben
- propylparaben
- other ingredients ending in -paraben

Day after day, we put chemicals on our skin, whether they are in lotion, makeup, shampoo, aftershave, or just plain soap. In fact, most women who wear makeup wear it for an average of fifteen hours a day, and many forget to wash it off before going to bed, giving the chemicals more time to leach into the bloodstream.

What we put on our skin matters, and that doesn't stop with those products we actively apply to our skin. Laundry detergents and bleach are regularly in contact with our skin via our clothes. Every day that we use chemical-based laundry detergent and bleach our whites, we are putting on a personal coat of chemicals. And every night when we go to bed and slip under the sheets, we rest against that same layer of potential chemical harm.

Whether we see the damage immediately, such as skin irritation, or the damage takes place over time on a cellular level, chemicals tax our immune system with every application.

With that said, however, imagine how much healthier your body would be, and how much better you would feel, if you eliminated as many of those harmful chemicals from your daily routine as possible?

Love Your Skin

The average woman uses twelve personal care products every day, and within these products are at least 168 different chemicals.

Men use fewer products, but they are still exposed to about eighty-five chemicals daily. This is a big area where making small changes and the choice of brands can make a big impact on your immune system.[22]

There are many healthy alternatives for a great many products out there today, thanks in large part to people who finally realized the long-term impact of using potential carcinogens, endocrine disruptors, and other toxins on our skin. Natural cosmetics, shampoos, deodorants, soaps, and laundry detergents are more affordable than they ever have been. In fact, plain, old, inexpensive hydrogen peroxide—that bubbly little antiseptic that Mom always poured on our cuts—is an excellent bleach alternative and stain remover.

This information may prompt you to immediately replace your products with safe ones; or as your current products run out, replace them with safer options. Either way, your body will thank you!

---

22 Dr. Joseph Mercola, "Women Put an Average of 168 Chemicals on Their Bodies Daily," www.mercola.com, May 13, 2015, accessed May 10, 2016, http://articles.mercola.com/sites/articles/archive/2015/05/13/toxic-chemicals-cosmetics.aspx.

Small Changes Make Big Impacts

Take an inventory of your personal care products. Which brands do you need to switch?

If this process feels overwhelming, visit www.NoToxinZone.com, enter your name and e-mail, and then fill out our "Health Awareness" survey and we will share the resources we personally use.

Positive Change

As you assess your home for all those things we've talked about in the past few chapters, don't let it overwhelm you. Even the littlest things, the smallest changes, can have a big impact. Switching out soda for water once a day, opening the windows instead of using artificial air fresheners—all of these small steps can have enormous impacts down the road.

"When 'I' is replaced by 'We' even 'Illness' becomes 'Wellness'."

CHAPTER 7
BE THE CHANGE

Small changes bring about big impacts. Just about every change we see in this world begins on an individual level because all it takes is one person to start a movement, one person with an idea or opinion, the courage to share it, and the drive to encourage others to follow.

Sadly, pain is often the catalyst for change. People may be bothered by pollution or morally outraged at the growing size of "trash continents" in our oceans, but until those things directly affect us, until they cause us pain, we are not as motivated to make changes. But when pain is real, it can be a powerful force.

Take Martin Luther King Jr. He was one man motivated by the pain he saw being caused by racial inequality, and he took his own steps to drive change and to encourage others to do the same. He added fire to the growing strength of the civil rights movement and became known for his approach of nonviolent, civil disobedience. His influence is still felt today as we continue to recognize Dr. King with memorials, posthumous awards, and days of recognition.

Just as the great pacifist and civil rights activist Mahatma Gandhi inspired Dr. King, we're also motivated to "be the change you wish to see in the world" because all it takes to start a great movement is one person.

The Wellness Movement

There is a wellness movement happening right now. It's about finding and treating the sources of illness as opposed to treating the symptoms, and we feel it is also about prevention.

Based on these theories, how can we make the shift from sick care to a culture of health? We need to create a movement, and as with any powerful movement, we're starting by doing our part. We begin with the choices we make for ourselves, and when others see that positive change in us, we provide the influence for others to make positive choices about their wellness.

Consider the movements created by great influencers such as Jillian Michaels, who broaches the subjects of fitness and weight loss; Dr. Mercola's alternative ideas about wellness; Joe Cross and his success in juicing his life back to health; Dr. Hyman and his ideas about reversing diabetes; Suzanne Somers telling women about aging. All of these influencers had the courage to share ideas that are different from the mainstream and, instead, focus on living a healthy, clean, toxin-free lifestyle.

Many people are already looking for the solutions that these advocates and many others are teaching. It's when enough people begin to adopt those ideas and take responsibility for their own health that we will begin to see the change we want to see in the world. But first we have to reach that tipping point.

Companies have a wonderful opportunity to bring wellness to the workplace and create tipping points, especially those we like to call the "early adapters." They tend to be ahead of the game when it comes to implementing new and innovative ideas in bettering our everyday health and are role models for those looking to improve health.

Take Google, for example. This company provides healthful benefits to its employees, such as energy pods that allow them to take a quick on-the-job power nap, free juice bars, and an open food pantry, as well as facilities to get their laundry done or take a shower without leaving the office.

Apple lets employees have thirty minutes a day to meditate, either in an in-office meditation room or through on-site yoga classes, and many companies such as Valero host "lunch-and-learn" events that focus on health-related issues such as cancer awareness.

All of these companies understand that keeping people healthy and happy in the first place will go a long way toward addressing the skyrocketing health-care costs facing this nation.

Companies such as Berkshire Hathaway even have the power to influence the health of entire cities. Omaha was recognized as one of America's healthiest cities due to the emphasis that Berkshire Hathaway has placed on personal health and wellness. Their wellness program provides employees with free access to tools and resources aimed at promoting long-term personal, physical, and financial health, rewarding successful participants with decreased health-care costs or monetary awards. As the CEO of Berkshire Hathaway, Warren Buffet, said, "There is no question that workplace wellness is worth it. The only question is whether you're going to do it today or tomorrow. If you keep saying you're going to do it tomorrow, you'll never do it."

Buffet's statement applies just as much to his company's wellness as it does to each of us as individuals seeking to be well. Taking it one step further, it's also been shown that happy people are also the most productive and innovative, so why not foster that attitude of healthfulness and happiness in the workplace?

Stress plays a huge role in turnover, with 42 percent of employees reporting, in 2014, that they left their job because of the stressful environment,[23] and another 35 percent considered changing jobs for the same reason.

On a more health-specific note, a 2011 Gallup poll found that 86 percent of employees are overweight and that they miss approximately 450 million extra days of work per year

---

23 "Dangerously Stressful Work Environments Force Workers to Seek New Employment," Monster, April 16, 2014, accessed May 10, 2016, http://www. monster.com/about/a/Dangerously-Stressful-Work-Environments-Force-Workers-to-Seek-New-Empl4162014-D3126696.

compared to healthy workers.[24] This results in an estimated cost to businesses of more than $153 billion annually.

We would say all of this constitutes a need for a change.

You Can Be the Change

Achieving change takes everyone doing his or her part, and nonprofit organizations are a great example of this because you can't do it on your own. You have to link up with other people! There's power in numbers, and when everyone starts to do the same thing, that's when the tipping point happens. The next thing you know, you have the change that you fought hard for.

Most people want to be a part of something greater than themselves, whether it's going to church, participating in a club, or supporting a nonprofit through volunteer and donation efforts. When people identify with a group for a specific reason, it evokes a sense of fulfillment that one simply can't achieve on one's own.

On a nonprofit level, organizations such as St. Baldrick's Foundation are making a big impact. Their head-shaving events are famous for bringing in large donations. Getting people to have their head shaved for childhood cancer research is no easy feat, yet their events grow larger each year.

---

24 Dan Witters and Sangeeta Agrawal, "Unhealthy U.S. Workers' Absenteeism Costs $153 Billion," Gallup, October 17, 2011, accessed May 10, 2016, http://www.gallup.com/poll/150026/unhealthy-workers-absenteeism-costs-153-billion.aspx.

The Max Love Project has also gained a lot of support in recent years. Max Wilford (SuperMax) was four years old when he was diagnosed with a rare and unusually aggressive form of a fairly common brain cancer. After five brain surgeries; two chemotherapy protocols; thirty radiation treatments; and integrative therapies, such as acupuncture, supplementation, Chinese herbs, and exercise, Max has thrived on a therapeutic superboosted ketogenic diet.

The Max Love project is inspired by Max's cancer journey and the tremendous benefits that he gained from this holistic, "whole-kid" approach to healing. Max Love believes that all superkids deserve every possible opportunity to conquer cancer. Their project is all about helping superkids thrive against the odds with fierce foods, whole-body wellness strategies, and integrative medicine. They are a community of hope dedicated to helping childhood cancer families beat the odds.

Participating in something that achieves a greater good is rewarding on an incredibly deep level, and getting behind a solid nonprofit is one of the best ways to get a movement going: plant the seed, spread the word, and start making those little steps toward the greater impact, that tipping point. Causes are like wildfire: they can ignite people to accomplish extraordinary things. And a good movement will go on no matter who is at the helm. That's the thing that keeps people tied together: that strong goal, that why.

Handing Hope . . . Our *Why*

For over a decade, we have taught others about wellness. Sharing the truth about toxins as they relate to our homes and bodies is our passion. After years of teaching the No Toxin Zone awareness program, we formed the nonprofit Handing H.O.P.E. with a twofold mission.

First, H.O.P.E. is an acronym for Helping Others through Prevention and Education. We offer wellness workshops that take a deeper dive into the No Toxin Zone program. We speak to churches, businesses, groups, and individuals about reducing their risk of cancer and living a healthy lifestyle. The more we spread our message of hope, the more people we can help to truly live well. We are being the change we want to see!

The second part of the Handing H.O.P.E. mission is Helping Others through Provision and Evangelism, which is how one of our biggest projects, the Lollipop Tree Project, originated.

Going through our own personal losses and battles with cancer, we felt the need to do something in the cancer community. Cancer is a big disease for children, and che-motherapy can literally leave a bad taste in your mouth. As parents, we can identify with the desire to give children a treat when they don't feel well. However, knowing that cancer thrives in a sugary environment, we needed to find a healthy sugar free alternative.

Our search brought us to Dr. John's Candies— lollipops and other treats that are sweetened with natural birch xylitol. Not only are the lollipops naturally sugar free, they are also kosher and free of gluten, soy, nuts, and dairy products, and they contain no artificial dyes. This makes them an ideal solution for any child in treatment, especially children with dietary restrictions. They even have a low-acid lollipop for children experiencing

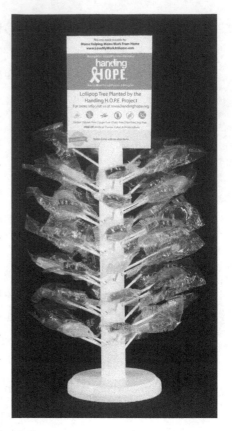

mouth sores as a result of chemotherapy treatment.

We donate or "plant" these lollipop trees in children's cancer clinics nationwide. We personally travel to the hospital to deliver the tree. We meet the staff and visit with the children. It is such a delight to see the smiles on even the sickest of children when they enjoy a lollipop from the tree. Those smiles and that comfort are why we do it. We want to bring hope and a smile to these children and show them how much we care about them and understand what they are going through.

We think about the parents as well and their need for hope and comfort. Next to each tree we leave literature to bring them encouragement. We also take prayer requests. The heart of our nonprofit is to continually sow seeds of hope for all who are in need.

The lollipop tree project doesn't stop with our initial visit to the hospital. We continue to "water" the trees by shipping lollipop refills monthly to each location we have planted a tree.

We have a big vision. We want to leave a legacy and give others the opportunity to do the same. We have found through our own losses that we do not want our loved ones to be forgotten. For this reason, we created a legacy program in which people can donate in memory of a friend or family member. We have found this to be a great way for those that have lost a loved one to extend their legacy.

If you are interested in supporting or learning more about the Lollipop Tree Project, please visit us at www.HandingHope.org.

Hope For Change

For Handing H.O.P.E. the Lollipop Tree Project is only the beginning of how we want to bring about change. The *goal* of the project is to provide a special treat to children who might otherwise not have been able to enjoy one, but the *purpose* was inspired by our desire to share information about the incredible value of clearing one's body and environment of common toxins.

For the Lollipop Tree Project, the toxin we fight is sugar, the nutrition-less substance that studies have linked to cancer. Beyond the lollipop project, we educate others about common physical and environmental pollutants, chemical-laced foods, toxic air and harmful engineered substances that we come in contact with everyday.

Knowledge is power. As we said at the beginning of *Be Well Assured*, "There is always hope." It is the resource we come back to time and again. It has been there for us every step of the way, and it's there for you too. Regardless of where you are or how you feel at this moment, know that in all things, there is hope.

CONCLUSION

BE WELL ASSURED, THERE IS HOPE

*For I know the plans I have for you. Plans to prosper you
and not to harm you, plans to give you hope and a future.*
—Jeremiah 29:11

Kim's Hope

Sometimes bad things happen to good people. I always
thought of myself as a good person. I had morals and faith in
God. I always lent a hand to those in need, and even though I
had endured divorce and other struggles in life, I still felt that
I'd strived for the good and positive in every day.

But then the words "your nodules are cancerous" rang in
my ears and never stopped. It took my breath away. My mind
was reeling, I couldn't breathe, and I couldn't cry. I tried to
listen to what the doctor was saying, but I couldn't hear his

words over the ringing of that statement. Afterward, I took my three-year-old daughter's hand, walked to the car, sat in the driver's seat, and wept. I mean, really wept. All I could think was, "God, is this it? You're going to take me out like this? Before I get to see my beautiful little daughter grow up?"

But then a peace came over me, and I felt God was saying that this disease wouldn't claim my life, that I would be able to use it to minister to others. He had a much bigger plan, and my cancer diagnosis was part of it.

Two years earlier, I had attended a wellness fair where I had met some people from a local cancer support center. I had picked up their brochure, thinking with my social work background I could help them by doing a support group or wellness workshop. That was the first time I felt that God was speaking to me to help those in the cancer community.

Fast-forward to the day of diagnosis. That day, when I got home from the doctor's office, that same brochure was sitting on top of a stack of papers on my dresser in my bedroom, even though I hadn't touched it or looked for it in two years.

I began to get this sense that all of this was happening for a reason. And that thought gave me hope.

The battle, however, was intense. There were days when I couldn't get out of bed, and I would just pray, read my Bible, and cry. I would ask God, "If you will just help me take a shower today, I will know you heard my prayer." And you know what? I would make it to that shower, even if I had to crawl.

Looking back at those dark and difficult days, God put so many provisions in my path. So many friends and family would come over just when I needed them. Yet still, there were days when I thought I was going to die. I wasn't afraid of death, but I wanted so badly to see my daughter grow up. I had almost died having her, and she was a miracle. God spared us both on the day she was born, and it was important to me to live, to be her mom, and to finish my life's purpose.

I struggled for months to regain my strength and regulate medications while, at the same time, trying to raise my daughter and run my household alone. There was no one there to help, so if I were sick at 2 a.m. and feeling horrible, it would just be God and me—but He never once let me down.

I honestly don't know what I would have done if I had had no faith, no one to cast my cares on. Fear would come over me at times, and anxiety attacks would wrack my body and mind, but day by day, I found hope in little things. I would play uplifting music, I kept a journal, I laughed, and I gave thanks.

Cancer changes your thoughts. On some mornings I would see the sunshine coming through my bedroom window and think, *You gave me another day. Thank you for that.*

I stopped sweating the small stuff because, in the grand scheme of life and death, those things really don't matter. Then, as time went on, I became stronger. I would still thank

Him for the day, but my prayers changed from asking Him to help me to asking Him, "What can I do for you today, Lord? Who can I bless or encourage?"

And He would bring people into my path. I found that helping others made my needs seem small, so I began to focus on helping others instead of focusing on my own struggles. After a while, those prayers evolved once again into, "How can I make an *impact* for you, Lord? What purpose do you have for me?"

After my battle, my best friend and coauthor Jen began losing those she loved to cancer. Her mom, her dad, and her best friend were all gone in a brief, two-year span. The grief she bore was indescribable.

There is something about watching someone you love bear pain so big that it feels as if it's physically hurting you too. I wanted it to end for her, but it didn't seem as if it ever would. But again, God was faithful. He made a way for her when there seemed there was no way at all. But because we trusted Him to help us and to help each other, we bore each other's burdens and gained strength and purpose in doing so.

Handing H.O.P.E. and this book were born of that strength—of my survival and Jen's greatest losses. God knit our passions, burdens, and trials into our purpose. Who better to empathize or encourage than one who has walked in the same shoes, who has found hope and can lead others to its source?

Jen's Hope

For three years I was buried in grief. First my father and then my mother and then my best friend all lost their battles with cancer, and it surprised me how much my body grieved physically. There were times, shortly after they passed, when I wasn't able to function. Grief is a heavy thing. Sometimes you feel you are going crazy. Those who have been through it know exactly what I am talking about. Talking to others who have been through grief gave me hope that I could move past this heavy, dark time and experience healing. My friend Rachelle Ferguson also lost both of her parents to cancer at young ages. She is an emerging voice related to grief recovery. I found talking with her and reading her blog, www.JoyAwaits. com, to be a great source of encouragement and strength.

If my parents and my best friend hadn't known the Lord, and if I hadn't believed that I would see them again one day because of their belief, I don't know if I could have ever climbed out of that grief. All I could do was cling to the truth that I would see them again. *If I live ten thousand more days*, I thought, *it's still temporary. Life is short and at the end of it, I'll be with the people I love. This is my hope.*

There are still days when grief tries to draw me back in. I have to fight that. In those moments, I think about my husband, my four children, and the fact that God has given me a ministry with a great purpose. The Lollipop Tree Project is a meaningful way in which I have been able to extend my parents' and best friend's legacy and honor them. In life, they were my biggest cheerleaders. They all loved children. I know they would be so proud of this project.

In the process of writing this book, I struggled for clarity one evening, after a day of ups and downs. I'd had a biopsy done that afternoon and had also received the video production for the story of "Handing Hope" that Kim and I had been working so hard on. I really wanted to call my parents and share the video with them, tell them about my day, and ask them for a prayer for my biopsy. For a moment the grief shook through me, and I found myself questioning God. *Here I am in the middle of writing a book to bring hope to those battling cancer and to help those looking to prevent cancer or continue surviving, and I could be facing my own diagnosis,* I thought.

I pleaded with God to speak to me, and in the midst of my prayer, I picked up my devotional *Jesus Calling* and read the chapter for the day. I got to only the second sentence and knew that God had heard my prayer. Let me share the devotional with you for that day. Maybe it will encourage you.

You are mine for all time; nothing can separate you from My Love. Since I invested my very life in you, BE WELL ASSURED that I will also take care of you. When your mind goes into neutral and your thoughts flow freely, you tend to feel anxious and alone. Your focus becomes problem solving. To get your mind back into gear, just turn toward Me, bringing yourself and your problems into My Presence.

Many problems vanish instantly in the Light of My Love because you realize you are never alone. Other problems may remain, but they become secondary to knowing Me and rejoicing in the relationship I so freely offer you. Each moment you can choose to practice my Presence or to practice the presence of problems.[25]

I felt the tears spilling down my cheeks as I read the words "BE WELL ASSURED," as only Kim, myself, and a small handful of close friends and family knew that was to be the title of this book. It absolutely amazes me that God inspired the author, Sarah Young, to pen those words on that particular day, years before I was really going to need it.

Our Hope for You

Our prayer is that we could be that inspiration for you, that whatever is going on in your life as you read this book, you are filled with hope when you finish reading it. We want you to know there is no circumstance too big for God. The truth is when you put your trust in Christ, He is able to change your circumstances or change your heart in those circumstances. He can be a source of complete peace, comfort, joy, and unconditional love. His word says He never leaves or

25 Sarah Young, Jesus Calling (Nashville, Tennessee: Thomas Nelson, 2004).

forsakes us. With that in mind, here are a few things that we want to share with you:

First, God loves you and has a plan for you!

The Bible says, "God so loved the world that He gave His one and only Son, [Jesus Christ], that whoever believes in Him shall not perish, but have eternal life" (John 3:16). Jesus said, "I came that they may have life and have it abundantly"—a complete life full of purpose (John 10:10).

We have all done, thought, or said bad things, which the Bible calls "sin." The Bible says, "All have sinned and fall short of the glory of God" (Romans 3:23). The result of sin is death, spiritual separation from God (Romans 6:23). Here is the good news. God sent his son to die for our sins! What that means for us is that he paid a price that we could not.

"God demonstrates his own love toward us, in that while we were yet sinners, Christ died for us" (Romans 5:8). But it didn't end with his death on the cross. He rose again and still lives!

We can't earn salvation; we are saved by God's grace when we surrender our hearts and put our faith in his son, Jesus Christ.

We need to turn from our sins, which is called repentance. What matters to him is the attitude of your heart, your honesty. Those who call upon the name of the Lord shall be saved (Romans 10:13).

Putting your trust in Christ and beginning a relationship with Him is simple. Quiet yourself and pour your heart out to God. Ask for forgiveness. Prayer is just talking to Him. If you seek Him, you will find Him, and He will reveal himself to you and renew your heart.

Our prayer is that you will *Be Well Assured* there is hope in this life and for eternity.

START BEING WELL ASSURED TODAY!

Connect with us for additional support and educational resources to implement positive and healthy changes in your own life.

HANDING HOPE ON FACEBOOK

Like us on Facebook, and follow our positive messages and updates.

WELLNESS WORKSHOPS

Host a wellness workshop for your church, company, community group or corporation. For more information, contact us at 800-689-1277.

DONATE OR JOIN OUR TEAM

To donate directly or learn more about fundraising, service project opportunities, and our shop and share program, visit us at www.HandingHope.org or e-mail us directly at admin@handinghope.org.

SHOP SMARTER AND SAFER

Watch our five-minute *No Toxin Zone* video, learn more about safer shopping solutions, and complete a Health Awareness Survey by visiting www.NoToxinZone.com.

FIND OUT YOUR BODY TOXICITY SCORE

To take our FREE "Know your Body's Toxicity Score" quiz, visit www.BeWellAssured.com.